FEMININE WELLNESS

A Guide to Hormonal Balance and Fasting Brilliance.

Author: Mae Walker

Editor: Crystal Abbott

Contents

INTRODUCTION...1

FEMININE WELLNESS...1

Historical Perspectives 3

Modern Perspectives 6

The Importance of Hormonal Balance 8

Impact of Hormonal Balance on Physical Health.........................11

Impact of Hormonal Balance on Mental Health...........................13

CHAPTER 1..17

The Foundation of Hormonal Health..17

Exploring the Endocrine System 19

Hormone Production and Release..24

Hormones and Their Functions 26

Key Hormones in Women...29

Interactions and Feedback Mechanisms 31

CHAPTER 2..34

Hormonal Imbalances in Women...34

Common Hormonal Issues...36

Polycystic Ovary Syndrome (PCOS) 40

Thyroid Disorders 42

Recognizing Symptoms 45

Physical Signs...49

Emotional and Behavioral Signs 53

CHAPTER 3..59

Nourishing Your Body for Hormonal Harmony.............................59

Nutrient-Rich Foods for Hormonal Balance 60

Essential Nutrients for Hormones 62

Foods to Support Hormone Production 66

The Role of Hydration in Wellness 69

Hydrating Foods and Beverages 76

CHAPTER 4 81

Fasting and Hormonal Brilliance 81

Intermittent Fasting 84

Different Approaches to Intermittent Fasting 86

Benefits and Risks of Intermittent Fasting 89

Fasting and Hormonal Regulation 93

Hormonal Responses to Fasting 96

CHAPTER 5 100

Tailoring Fasting to the Female Body 100

Hormonal Considerations for Fasting 102

Menstrual Cycle and Fasting 105

Fasting during Pregnancy and Lactation 107

Creating a Personalized Fasting Plan 110

Self-Help Questions 114

INTRODUCTION

FEMININE WELLNESS

Women increasingly embrace empowerment and are willing to engage in open conversations regarding intimate health matters in various settings. As a result of evolving societal attitudes, there is a growing awareness among women regarding feminine wellness. There has been a notable shift in societal attitudes towards women's vaginal health in recent years. Previously stigmatized, women now exhibit a greater level of comfort when discussing issues related to this area of their well-being. Furthermore, there is an increased recognition among women that intimate health and skincare require diligent care and attention. For example, the vaginal pH level significantly impacts overall health and well-being. Maintaining a balanced pH can help prevent infections, enhance energy levels, and address digestive health concerns like bloating.

Feminine wellness encompasses a holistic approach to health, focusing on women's unique needs and experiences. It goes beyond the traditional understanding of health and delves into the intricate interplay of physical, mental, and emotional well-being. Here's a detailed exploration of key aspects within the realm of feminine wellness:

I. Physical Health:

- *Hormonal Balance:* The delicate dance of hormones is at the core of feminine wellness. Achieving and maintaining hormonal balance is crucial for a woman's overall health. This involves understanding the endocrine system, recognizing common hormonal issues, and adopting nourishing habits to support optimal hormone levels.

- ***Nutrition:*** Nourishing the body with the proper nutrients is a cornerstone of feminine wellness. This includes focusing on nutrient-rich foods that support hormonal health and hydration practices that promote overall well-being.

- ***Fasting Brilliance:*** Intermittent fasting, when tailored to the female body, can be a powerful tool for hormonal regulation. It's about understanding the nuances of fasting and creating personalized plans that align with women's unique hormonal considerations.

2. Mental and Emotional Well-being:

- ***Mind-Body Connection:*** Feminine wellness recognizes the profound link between mental and physical health. Stress management, mindfulness practices, and emotional well-being are integral components. Addressing stressors and fostering emotional resilience contribute significantly to overall wellness.

- ***Exercise and Balance:*** Physical activity is not just about fitness; it plays a pivotal role in hormonal balance. The proper compensation for training can positively influence endorphins, stress hormones, and sex hormones. Tailoring exercise routines to individual needs is critical.

3. Lifelong Approach:

- ***Adolescence to Menopause:*** Feminine wellness takes a lifespan approach, acknowledging the changing dynamics of hormones from youth through menopause. Special considerations for each stage, including fertility and post-menopausal health, are woven into the fabric of this approach.

4. Practical Tips and Everyday Balance:

- *Lifestyle Changes:* Implementing sustainable lifestyle changes is emphasized for lasting wellness. This includes optimizing sleep, addressing environmental factors, and creating habits that support hormonal balance.

- *Integration into Daily Life:* Feminine wellness isn't a temporary endeavor; it's about seamlessly integrating well-being into daily life. From meal planning to stress management techniques, the goal is to make wellness a part of one's routine.

5. Empowerment:

- *Taking Charge:* A central theme in feminine wellness is empowerment. It encourages women to actively understand their bodies, make informed choices, and advocate for their health. This empowerment forms the foundation for a journey towards hormonal brilliance.

Historical Perspectives

Understanding feminine wellness requires a journey through history, tracing the evolving perceptions and practices related to women's health. The treatment of women's well-being has been shaped by cultural, societal, and medical contexts, reflecting progress and challenges.

I. Ancient Wisdom:

- In ancient civilizations, including ancient Greece, China, and India, there existed a recognition of the interconnectedness of health's physical, mental, and emotional aspects. Women were often regarded as the bearers of life, and various cultural practices and rituals were dedicated to honoring and preserving their well-being.

- Traditional medicine systems, such as Ayurveda and Traditional Chinese Medicine, acknowledged the importance of hormonal balance and the role of nutrition in supporting women's health.

2. Middle Ages and Renaissance:

- The Middle Ages witnessed a shift in medical practices, with a more systematic approach to understanding the human body. However, societal views often constrained women's roles to those of mothers and caretakers, impacting the discourse on their health.

- The Renaissance period brought about renewed interest in human anatomy and health. Yet, discussions around women's health were often influenced by societal norms and sometimes veiled in misconceptions.

3. 18th to 19th Century:

- The 18th and 19th centuries marked a significant transformation in understanding women's health. The emergence of gynecology led to more systematic examinations of reproductive health. However, cultural taboos and limited medical knowledge still posed challenges.

- The Victorian era, characterized by rigid social norms, brought about progress and repression. Discussions around women's health became more structured, but the prevailing societal attitudes sometimes hindered open dialogue.

4. 20th Century to Present:

- The 20th century witnessed substantial advancements in medicine and women's rights. The development of hormonal contraceptives and breakthroughs in reproductive health marked milestones. However, societal expectations and stereotypes persisted, influencing medical research and healthcare practices.

- In recent decades, there has been a growing recognition of the unique aspects of women's health beyond reproductive concerns. The field of feminine wellness has expanded to encompass a holistic view, addressing hormonal balance, mental health, and lifestyle factors.

5. Cultural and Global Perspectives:

- Cultural diversity plays a vital role in shaping perspectives on feminine wellness. Indigenous practices, traditional rituals, and community support systems contribute to a rich tapestry of approaches to women's health worldwide.

- Global movements advocating for women's rights and health equity have led to increased awareness and initiatives addressing issues such as maternal health, access to education, and healthcare disparities.

In the contemporary context, feminine wellness emerges as a dynamic and evolving concept influenced by historical legacies and modern insights. It reflects the ongoing journey to understand, celebrate, and optimize the well-being of women across cultures and generations.

Modern Perspectives

In the 21st century, the landscape of feminine wellness has evolved significantly, reflecting a more nuanced and inclusive understanding of women's health. Modern perspectives on feminine wellness encompass a holistic approach beyond traditional medical paradigms, emphasizing empowerment, individualization, and integrating diverse elements.

I. Holistic Well-being:

- **Physical Health:** Modern perspectives recognize the multifaceted nature of women's health, extending beyond reproductive concerns. There is an emphasis on holistic well-being, incorporating aspects such as hormonal balance, nutrition, and fitness.

- **Mental and Emotional Health:** Acknowledging the intimate connection between psychological and physical health is central. Addressing stress, promoting mindfulness, and fostering emotional resilience are integral to modern feminine wellness.

2. Empowerment and Informed Choices:

- **Education and Awareness:** Women are encouraged to participate proactively in their health journey. Access to information and education empowers them to make informed choices regarding their bodies, healthcare decisions, and overall well-being.

- **Advocacy for Women's Rights:** Modern perspectives align with movements advocating for women's rights, recognizing the importance of healthcare equity, access to education, and the dismantling of societal barriers that impact women's health.

3. Personalization of Care:

- **Individualized Approaches:** Modern feminine wellness recognizes the uniqueness of each woman. Health recommendations and interventions are increasingly tailored to individual needs, considering genetics, lifestyle, and personal preferences.

- **Technology and Data:** Advancements in technology, including wearable devices and health apps, enable women to track and understand their bodies more effectively. This data-driven approach facilitates personalized health management.

4. Inclusive Discussions:

- **Breaking Taboos:** Modern perspectives encourage open and inclusive discussions around women's health. Breaking taboos related to menstruation, menopause, and reproductive health fosters a culture of understanding and support.

- **Diverse Experiences:** Recognizing and respecting the diverse experiences of women, including those from different cultural backgrounds and identities, is a crucial aspect of modern feminine wellness.

5. Integrative and Preventive Health:

- **Integrative Medicine:** Integrating conventional medicine with complementary and alternative approaches is gaining prominence. Practices like acupuncture, herbal medicine, and mind-body therapies are explored for their potential benefits in women's health.

- **Preventive Measures:** There is a growing emphasis on preventative healthcare. Lifestyle modifications, including diet, exercise, and stress management, are essential to maintaining optimal feminine wellness.

6. Global Collaboration:

- **Health Equity:** Modern perspectives on feminine wellness advocate for global health equity. Initiatives and collaborations address healthcare disparities, ensuring women worldwide have access to quality healthcare and education.

- **Research and Innovation:** Ongoing research and innovation contribute to a deeper understanding of women's health issues. Advances in medical technology and treatments continue to shape modern approaches to feminine wellness.

The Importance of Hormonal Balance

Hormonal balance is a fundamental aspect of overall health and well-being, pivotal in numerous physiological processes within the body. Hormones act as messengers, regulating everything from metabolism and mood to reproductive cycles and immune function. Understanding and maintaining hormonal balance is crucial for several reasons:

I. Regulation of Vital Functions:

- **Metabolism:** Hormones, such as insulin and thyroid hormones, play a crucial role in regulating metabolism. Imbalances can contribute to weight issues, fatigue, and metabolic disorders.

- **Reproductive Health:** Hormonal balance is essential for menstrual regularity, fertility, and a healthy pregnancy.

Disruptions can lead to polycystic ovary syndrome (PCOS) or fertility issues.

2. Emotional and Mental Well-being:

- **Neurotransmitters:** Hormones influence neurotransmitters that regulate mood and emotions. Balanced hormones contribute to mental well-being, while imbalances may lead to mood swings, anxiety, or depression.

- **Stress Hormones:** Cortisol, the primary stress hormone, impacts emotional resilience. Chronic stress and hormonal imbalance can create a cycle of emotional and physical health challenges.

3. Bone Health:

- **Calcium Regulation:** Hormones like estrogen are crucial in maintaining bone density. Declining estrogen levels, especially during menopause, can contribute to bone loss and osteoporosis.

4. Immune System Function:

- **Cytokines:** Hormones influence the production and activity of immune system components. Imbalances can affect immune function, making the body more susceptible to infections or autoimmune conditions.

5. Sleep Patterns:

- **Melatonin:** Hormones regulate the sleep-wake cycle. Disruptions in hormonal balance, particularly melatonin levels, can lead to sleep disturbances and insomnia.

6. Skin Health:

- **Collagen Production:** Hormones contribute to collagen production, which maintains skin elasticity. Hormonal imbalances may contribute to skin issues such as acne or premature aging.

7. Blood Sugar Regulation:

- **Insulin:** Hormones like insulin regulate blood sugar levels. Imbalances can lead to insulin resistance and contribute to the development of diabetes.

8. Cardiovascular Health:

- **Blood Pressure:** Hormones influence blood pressure regulation. Imbalances may contribute to hypertension and cardiovascular issues.

9. Cognitive Function:

- **Brain Health:** Hormones affect cognitive function, memory, and concentration. Hormonal imbalances may affect cognitive performance.

10. Adaptation to Stress:

- **Adrenal Hormones:** Hormones produced by the adrenal glands, such as cortisol, help the body respond to stress. Prolonged stress and hormonal imbalance can lead to adrenal fatigue.

Achieving and maintaining hormonal balance involves a combination of lifestyle factors, including a balanced diet, regular exercise, stress management, and, in some cases, medical interventions. Regular monitoring of hormonal health is essential for early detection and intervention in cases of imbalance.

In essence, hormonal balance is not just about reproductive health; it is a cornerstone of overall well-being, influencing various physiological systems. Prioritizing hormonal health contributes to a vibrant, energetic, and emotionally resilient life.

Impact of Hormonal Balance on Physical Health

Maintaining hormonal balance is crucial for optimal physical health, as hormones act as messengers that regulate various physiological processes within the body. Disruptions in hormonal equilibrium can profoundly affect multiple systems, leading to various health issues. Here's a closer look at how hormonal balance influences physical health:

I. Metabolic Health:

- **Insulin and Glucose Regulation:** Hormonal balance, particularly insulin sensitivity, is essential for regulating blood sugar levels. Imbalances can contribute to insulin resistance, metabolic syndrome, and the development of type 2 diabetes.

- **Thyroid Hormones:** Thyroid hormones influence metabolism. Imbalances, such as hypothyroidism or hyperthyroidism, can impact energy levels, weight, and overall metabolic function.

2. Reproductive Health:

- **Menstrual Regularity:** Hormonal balance is crucial for the regularity of menstrual cycles. Imbalances, such as those in polycystic ovary syndrome (PCOS) or hormonal contraceptives, can affect reproductive health.

- **Pregnancy and Fertility:** Balanced hormones are essential for fertility and a healthy pregnancy. Imbalances may contribute to fertility issues, miscarriages, or complications during pregnancy.

3. Bone Health:

- **Estrogen and Calcium Regulation:** Estrogen plays a vital role in maintaining bone density by regulating calcium absorption. Hormonal imbalances significantly decrease estrogen during menopause, which can lead to bone loss and osteoporosis.

4. Cardiovascular Function:

- **Blood Pressure:** Hormones influence blood vessel constriction and dilation, affecting blood pressure. Imbalances may contribute to hypertension and increase the risk of cardiovascular diseases.

- **Cholesterol Levels:** Hormones impact lipid metabolism. Imbalances can contribute to unfavorable lipid profiles, increasing the risk of heart disease.

5. Immune System Function:

- **Cytokine Production:** Hormones influence the production and activity of immune system components. Imbalances can affect immune function, making the body more susceptible to infections or autoimmune conditions.

6. Weight Management:

- **Leptin and Ghrelin:** Hormones like leptin and ghrelin affect appetite regulation. Imbalances may contribute to overeating, weight gain, or difficulties in weight management.

7. Energy Levels:

- **Adrenal Hormones:** Hormones produced by the adrenal glands, including cortisol and adrenaline, influence energy levels. Chronic stress and hormonal imbalances can lead to fatigue and adrenal fatigue.

8. Skin Health:

- **Androgens and Estrogen:** Hormones influence skin health by regulating oil production and collagen levels. Imbalances can contribute to skin issues such as acne or premature aging.

9. Thermoregulation:

- **Estrogen and Menopause:** Hormonal changes during menopause, particularly the decline in estrogen, can impact thermoregulation, leading to hot flashes and night sweats.

10. Physical Performance:

- **Growth Hormone:** Hormones like growth hormone play a role in muscle growth and repair. Imbalances may impact physical performance and recovery.

Achieving and maintaining hormonal balance involves lifestyle factors such as a balanced diet, regular exercise, stress management, and, in some cases, medical interventions. Regular monitoring of hormonal health is essential for early detection and intervention in cases of imbalance.

Impact of Hormonal Balance on Mental Health

Hormonal balance is crucial in mental health, influencing mood, cognition, and emotional well-being. The intricate interplay between hormones and the brain's neurotransmitter systems underscores the significance of hormonal equilibrium for mental and emotional stability. Here's a closer look at how hormonal balance impacts mental health:

1. Neurotransmitter Regulation:

- **Serotonin and Dopamine:** Hormonal balance is intricately connected to regulating neurotransmitters such as serotonin and dopamine. Imbalances can affect mood regulation, contributing to conditions like depression and anxiety.

2. Stress Response:

- **Cortisol:** The stress hormone cortisol, produced by the adrenal glands, is crucial for the body's response to stress. However, chronic tension and elevated cortisol levels can impact mental health, leading to anxiety, irritability, and cognitive decline.

3. Estrogen and Mood:

- **Menstrual Cycle:** Fluctuations in estrogen levels during the menstrual cycle can influence mood. Some women may experience changes in mood, irritability, or heightened emotional sensitivity during specific phases of the process.

- **Menopause:** The decline in estrogen during menopause is associated with an increased risk of mood disorders such as depression and anxiety.

4. GABA and Hormonal Balance:

- **Gamma-Aminobutyric Acid (GABA):** GABA is an inhibitory neurotransmitter that calms the nervous system. Hormonal imbalances can affect GABA levels, contributing to anxiety and insomnia.

5. Thyroid Hormones and Cognitive Function:

- **Thyroid Disorders:** Imbalances in thyroid hormones, such as hypothyroidism or hyperthyroidism, can impact cognitive function, leading to symptoms like brain fog, memory issues, and difficulty concentrating.

6. Reproductive Hormones and Emotional Well-being:

- **Progesterone:** Fluctuations in progesterone levels, particularly during the menstrual cycle, can influence emotional well-being. Some women may experience changes in mood, anxiety, or even depression during certain phases.

7. Cognitive Health and Aging:

- **Estrogen and Cognitive Decline:** Estrogen has neuroprotective effects, and its decline during menopause is associated with an increased risk of cognitive decline and conditions like Alzheimer's disease.

8. Sleep and Mental Health:

- **Melatonin:** Hormones, including melatonin, regulate sleep-wake cycles. Disruptions in hormonal balance, such as those seen in sleep disorders, can impact mental health by affecting mood, cognitive function, and overall well-being.

9. Hormonal Contraceptives and Mood:

- **Synthetic Hormones:** Some individuals may experience mood or emotional well-being changes as a side effect of hormonal contraceptives. Individuals need to be aware of potential impacts on mental health when considering contraceptive options.

10. Stress Resilience:

- **Adrenal Hormones:** Hormones produced by the adrenal glands, including cortisol and adrenaline, influence the body's stress response. Chronic stress and hormonal imbalances can impact stress resilience, leading to mental health challenges.

CHAPTER 1

The Foundation of Hormonal Health.

In the intricate symphony of the human body, the endocrine system takes center stage as the conductor of hormonal harmony. The foundation of hormonal health is laid upon a deep understanding of this complex system that orchestrates the delicate dance of hormones, guiding every facet of our physical and mental well-being.

1. The Endocrine System: An Intricate Network:

- The endocrine system is at the core of hormonal health— a network of glands that produce and release hormones into the bloodstream. These hormones act as messengers, traveling to target organs and tissues to regulate various physiological processes.

- Glands such as the pituitary, thyroid, adrenal, and ovaries (in females) play pivotal roles in this system. Each gland has unique responsibilities, contributing to hormones' balance and coordination.

2. Hormones: Messengers of Regulation:

- Hormones are the silent conductors of the body's orchestra. From insulin and cortisol to estrogen and testosterone, these chemical messengers wield immense influence over metabolism, reproductive cycles, mood, and more.

- Understanding the functions of critical hormones is essential. Insulin, for example, regulates blood sugar, while cortisol responds to stress. Estrogen and progesterone guide the menstrual cycle and impact fertility.

3. Feedback Mechanisms: Balancing the Score:

- Hormonal balance is not a static state; it's a dynamic equilibrium maintained by intricate feedback mechanisms. When hormone levels fluctuate, feedback loops activate to bring the system back to balance.

- For instance, the hypothalamus and pituitary gland work in tandem to regulate thyroid hormone production. Feedback loops ensure the right amount of hormones is released at the right time.

4. Common Hormonal Issues: Recognizing the Discord:

- Understanding hormonal imbalances is crucial for maintaining health. Common issues such as hypothyroidism, hyperthyroidism, insulin resistance, and polycystic ovary syndrome (PCOS) can disrupt the symphony, leading to various health challenges.

- Recognizing the signs and symptoms of hormonal issues—irregular menstrual cycles, fatigue, or mood changes—empowers individuals to seek timely intervention.

5. Nourishing the Endocrine Ecosystem:

- The foundation of hormonal health extends to lifestyle choices, especially nutrition. Nutrient-dense foods provide the raw materials necessary for hormone production and balance.

- Balanced nutrition supports the endocrine ecosystem, ensuring that glands have the essential vitamins and minerals for optimal function. Nutrients like omega-3 fatty acids, zinc, and vitamin D are vital for hormonal health.

6. Holistic Wellness for Hormonal Harmony:

- The foundation of hormonal health goes beyond isolated interventions. Holistic wellness practices, including stress management, regular physical activity, and sufficient sleep, contribute to hormonal harmony.

- Stress, in particular, can act as a disruptor, influencing the release of cortisol and impacting other hormonal axes. Mind-body practices like meditation and yoga play a vital role in stress reduction.

Exploring the Endocrine System

The endocrine system, a marvel of intricate communication and regulation, is the silent conductor orchestrating the harmonious balance of hormones within the human body. This exploration into the endocrine system unveils its components, functions, and pivotal role in maintaining the delicate equilibrium of physiological processes.

I. Glands of Influence:

- **Pituitary Gland:** Often referred to as the "master gland," the pituitary gland controls the function of other endocrine glands. It secretes hormones that regulate growth, thyroid function, and reproductive processes.

- **Thyroid Gland:** The thyroid gland in the neck produces hormones that govern metabolism. Thyroid hormones influence energy expenditure, body temperature, and the utilization of nutrients.

- **Adrenal Glands:** Positioned atop the kidneys, adrenal glands produce hormones like cortisol and adrenaline. These hormones are integral to the body's stress response, regulating energy and the fight-or-flight response.

- **Pancreas:** Essential for glucose regulation, the pancreas produces insulin and glucagon. Insulin facilitates glucose uptake by cells, while glucagon releases glucose into the bloodstream when needed.

- **Ovaries (in females) and Testes (in males):** Responsible for producing sex hormones—estrogen and progesterone in females and testosterone in males. These hormones govern reproductive processes and secondary sexual characteristics.

2. Hormones: Messengers of the Endocrine Symphony:

- **Insulin:** Released by the pancreas, insulin regulates blood sugar levels by facilitating glucose uptake by cells for energy.

- **Cortisol:** Produced by the adrenal glands, cortisol responds to stress, influencing metabolism, immune function, and the sleep-wake cycle.

- **Thyroid Hormones (T3 and T4):** Secreted by the thyroid gland, these hormones play a central role in regulating metabolism, energy production, and body temperature.

- **Estrogen and Progesterone:** Produced by the ovaries, these hormones regulate the menstrual cycle, support pregnancy, and contribute to overall reproductive health.

- **Testosterone:** Produced by the testes, testosterone influences male reproductive function, muscle mass, bone density, and secondary sexual characteristics.

3. Communication through Feedback Loops:

- The endocrine system operates through feedback loops that maintain hormonal balance. When hormone levels deviate from the desired range, feedback mechanisms activate to adjust secretion.

- For example, the hypothalamus and pituitary gland work together to regulate thyroid hormone levels. If thyroid hormone levels are low, the hypothalamus releases thyrotropin-releasing hormone (TRH), stimulating the pituitary to release thyroid-stimulating hormone (TSH), prompting the thyroid to produce more hormones.

4. Hormonal Imbalances: Disruptions in the Harmony:

- Hormonal imbalances can lead to various health issues. For instance, an underactive thyroid (hypothyroidism) can result in fatigue, weight gain, and cold intolerance. Conversely, an overactive thyroid (hyperthyroidism) can cause weight loss, irritability, and heat sensitivity.

- Conditions like diabetes, characterized by insulin resistance or insufficient insulin production, showcase the impact of hormonal imbalances on blood sugar regulation.

5. The Dance of Hormones in Reproductive Health:

- The endocrine system plays a crucial role in reproductive health. The menstrual cycle, controlled by hormones like estrogen and progesterone, is a testament to the orchestration of complex hormonal events.

- Pregnancy involves a delicate interplay of hormones to support fetal development and maintain a healthy pregnancy.

The endocrine system, composed of various glands scattered strategically throughout the body, is the conductor of a symphony, orchestrating the intricate dance of hormones that regulate physiological processes. Here's an overview of the key players in this hormonal symphony:

1. Pituitary Gland: The Master Conductor:

- *Location:* Nestled at the base of the brain in a bony structure called the sella turcica.

- *Function:* Often referred to as the "master gland," the pituitary gland regulates the activity of other endocrine glands. It produces growth hormone, thyroid-stimulating hormone, and gonadotropins that influence growth, metabolism, and reproductive processes.

2. Thyroid Gland: Metabolic Maestro:

- *Location:* Found in the neck, wrapped around the trachea.

- *Function:* Produces thyroid hormones (T3 and T4) that are central in regulating metabolism, energy production, and body temperature. Also, it secretes calcitonin, which is involved in calcium regulation.

3. Adrenal Glands: Stress Response Virtuosos:

- *Location:* Situated atop each kidney.

- *Function:* Release hormones such as cortisol and adrenaline in response to stress. These hormones influence metabolism, immune function, and the body's fight-or-flight response.

4. **Pancreas: Glucose Regulator:**

- *Location:* Behind the stomach, nestled between the spleen and the small intestine.

- *Function:* Produces insulin and glucagon, crucial for regulating blood sugar levels. Insulin facilitates glucose uptake by cells, while glucagon releases glucose into the bloodstream when needed.

5. **Ovaries (in Females): Regulators of Reproduction:**

- *Location:* Located in the pelvis.

- *Function:* Produce hormones such as estrogen and progesterone that regulate the menstrual cycle, support pregnancy, and influence secondary sexual characteristics.

6. **Testes (in Males): Conductors of Masculine Characteristics:**

- *Location:* Housed in the scrotum.

- *Function:* Produce testosterone, influencing the male reproductive process, muscle mass, bone density, and secondary sexual characteristics.

7. **Hypothalamus: The Maestro's Assistant:**

- *Location:* Situated at the base of the brain.

- *Function:* Acts as a crucial link between the nervous and endocrine systems. It releases and inhibits hormones that signal the pituitary gland to remove or inhibit the production of certain hormones.

8. **Parathyroid Glands: Calcium Conductors:**

- *Location:* Four small glands located on the thyroid gland.

- *Function:* Regulate calcium levels in the blood by producing parathyroid hormone (PTH), which influences calcium release from bones and absorption in the intestines.

9. Thymus: Immune System Orchestrator:

- *Location:* Located behind the sternum.

- *Function:* Plays a role in immune system development and process, particularly in early life. Produces hormones that support the maturation of T cells, crucial for immune defense.

Hormone Production and Release

Like a finely tuned orchestra, the endocrine system relies on precise signals, hormone production, and release timings. Each gland plays a unique instrument in this symphony, contributing to the harmony of physiological processes. Let's explore how hormones are crafted and conducted through the intricate dance of production and release:

1. Initiation: The Maestro Hypothalamus:

- The overture to hormone release begins in the hypothalamus, nestled at the base of the brain. This master conductor senses the body's needs and initiates hormonal responses by producing releasing and inhibiting hormones.

2. Command to the Pituitary Gland: The Master's Cue:

- The hypothalamus dispatches releasing or inhibiting hormones to the pituitary gland, positioned nearby. The pituitary gland often hailed as the "master gland," takes these cues and responds by releasing its own set of hormones.

3. **Pituitary Hormones: Signaling the Orchestra:**

- The pituitary gland secretes hormones like thyroid-stimulating hormone (TSH), adrenocorticotropic hormone (ACTH), growth hormone (GH), and more. Each hormone signals a specific target gland to orchestrate the production of its unique hormones.

4. **Target Gland Activation: Specialized Players Take the Stage:**

- Each target gland, the thyroid, adrenal, or reproductive glands, receives the pituitary's cue and begins producing its characteristic hormones. For example, the thyroid gland releases thyroid hormones (T3 and T4) in response to TSH.

5. **Feedback Mechanisms: The Harmonic Loop:**

- As hormone levels reach the desired range, feedback mechanisms come into play. The target gland hormones send signals back to the hypothalamus and pituitary, indicating whether more or less stimulation is needed. This feedback loop maintains the delicate balance of hormones.

6. **Transportation: Hormones on the Move:**

- Once released, hormones travel through the bloodstream to reach target cells or organs. Their specific chemical structure allows them to bind to receptors on these target cells, initiating a cascade of biological responses.

7. **Effect on Target Cells: Harmonizing Cellular Responses:**

- Hormones act as messengers, delivering instructions to target cells. The response varies based on the type of hormone and the receptors present in the cell. For example, insulin prompts cells to take up glucose, while cortisol influences metabolism and immune function.

8. **Metabolism and Elimination: The Finale:**

- Hormones affect cellular functions, influencing metabolism, growth, immune responses, and more. Once their role is fulfilled, hormones are metabolized or eliminated, completing the cycle until the next cue from the hypothalamus initiates the symphony anew.

9. **Circadian Rhythms: The Day-Night Sonata:**

- Hormone production follows circadian rhythms, synchronized with the body's internal clock. For instance, cortisol levels peak in the morning, helping to wake the body and decline at night to facilitate sleep.

Hormones and Their Functions

With its array of hormones, the endocrine system orchestrates a symphony of physiological responses, influencing everything from metabolism to mood. Let's explore some essential hormones and their multifaceted roles in maintaining the delicate balance of the body:

1. **Insulin: The Glucose Maestro:**

- *Source:* Produced by the pancreas.

- *Function:* Regulates blood sugar levels by facilitating glucose uptake into cells, where it's used for energy. Insufficient insulin or insulin resistance can lead to diabetes.

2. Glucagon: Glucose Reservoir Caller:

- *Source:* Also produced by the pancreas.

- *Function:* Stimulates the release of glucose from the liver, increasing blood sugar levels when needed, such as between meals or during physical activity.

3. Cortisol: The Stress Symphony Conductor:

- *Source:* Produced by the adrenal glands.

- *Function:* Regulates the body's response to stress, influencing metabolism, immune function, and the sleep-wake cycle. Chronic elevation of cortisol due to prolonged stress can have various health implications.

4. Adrenaline (Epinephrine): The Fight-or-Flight Virtuoso:

- *Source:* Also produced by the adrenal glands.

- *Function:* Triggers the body's "fight-or-flight" response in stressful situations, increasing heart rate, dilating airways, and redirecting blood flow to vital organs.

5. Thyroid Hormones (T3 and T4): Metabolic Choreographers:

- *Source:* Produced by the thyroid gland.

- *Function:* Regulate metabolism, energy production, and body temperature. Imbalances can lead to conditions such as hypothyroidism or hyperthyroidism.

6. Estrogen and Progesterone: Reproductive Harmony Directors:

- *Source:* Produced by the ovaries in females.

- *Function:* Regulate the menstrual cycle, support pregnancy, and influence secondary sexual characteristics. Estrogen also plays a role in bone health.

7. Testosterone: Masculine Essence Composer:

- *Source:* Produced by the testes in males.

- *Function:* Influences male reproductive function, muscle mass, bone density, and the development of secondary sexual characteristics.

8. Growth Hormone: Architect of Growth and Repair:

- *Source:* Produced by the pituitary gland.

- *Function:* Stimulates growth, cell reproduction, and regeneration. Plays a crucial role in childhood growth and ongoing tissue repair.

9. Melatonin: Sleep Serenade Conductor:

- *Source:* Produced by the pineal gland in response to darkness.

- *Function:* Regulates the sleep-wake cycle and influences circadian rhythms. Melatonin supplements are often used to aid sleep.

10. Parathyroid Hormone (PTH): Calcium Balancer:

- *Source:* Produced by the parathyroid glands.

- *Function:* Regulates calcium levels in the blood by influencing calcium release from bones and absorption in the intestines.

11. Aldosterone: Sodium and Water Maestro:

- *Source:* Produced by the adrenal glands.

- *Function:* Regulates sodium and water balance in the body, influencing blood pressure and electrolyte levels.

12. **Leptin: The Satiety Composer:**

- *Source:* Produced by fat cells.

- *Function:* Signals to the brain that the body has enough fat stores, influencing appetite and metabolism.

Understanding these hormones and their functions provides a glimpse into the complex interplay that governs the body's intricate processes. Like notes in a symphony, each hormone contributes to the harmonious functioning of the body's physiological orchestra.

Key Hormones in Women

The hormonal landscape in women is a dynamic and intricate symphony where various hormones play distinct roles in regulating reproductive health, mood, and overall well-being. Let's explore some essential hormones in women and their functions:

1. **Estrogen: The Orchestrator of Feminine Vitality:**

- *Source:* Primarily produced by the ovaries.

- *Function:* Governs the menstrual cycle, supports pregnancy, and influences secondary sexual characteristics. Estrogen also plays a role in bone health and cardiovascular function.

2. **Progesterone: The Menstrual Cycle Harmonizer:**

- *Source:* Produced by the ovaries (specifically, the corpus luteum) and later by the placenta during pregnancy.

- *Function:* Works in tandem with estrogen to regulate the menstrual cycle. In pregnancy, progesterone supports the maintenance of the uterine lining and prevents contractions.

3. Testosterone: The Androgenic Influence:

- *Source:* Produced in small amounts by the ovaries and adrenal glands.

- *Function:* While often associated with males, women also produce testosterone. It contributes to libido, energy levels, and muscle and bone mass maintenance.

4. FSH (Follicle-Stimulating Hormone): Initiator of Ovulation:

- *Source:* Secreted by the pituitary gland.

- *Function:* Stimulates the development of follicles in the ovaries, leading to the maturation of eggs. FSH is crucial for the initiation of ovulation.

5. LH (Luteinizing Hormone): Ovulation Maestro:

- *Source:* Also produced by the pituitary gland.

- *Function:* Triggers ovulation, the release of a mature egg from the ovaries. LH surge is a vital indicator of the fertile window in the menstrual cycle.

6. Prolactin: The Lactation Conductor:

- *Source:* Produced by the pituitary gland.

- *Function:* Stimulates milk production in the mammary glands during pregnancy and lactation. Elevated prolactin levels can inhibit ovulation.

7. Gonadotropins: FSH and LH Duo:

- *Source:* Secreted by the pituitary gland.

- *Function:* FSH and LH, collectively known as gonadotropins, regulate the menstrual cycle and support fertility by orchestrating the ovarian and uterine processes.

8. **Cortisol: The Stress Response Leader:**

- *Source:* Produced by the adrenal glands.

- *Function:* Regulates the body's response to stress, influences metabolism, and can impact the menstrual cycle. Chronic stress can lead to disruptions in cortisol levels.

9. **Thyroid Hormones (T3 and T4): Metabolic Choreographers:**

- *Source:* Produced by the thyroid gland.

- *Function:* Regulate metabolism, energy production, and body temperature. Thyroid hormones can influence the menstrual cycle and fertility.

10. **Melatonin: The Sleep-Wake Maestro:**

- *Source:* Produced by the pineal gland in response to darkness.

- *Function:* Regulates the sleep-wake cycle and influences circadian rhythms. Melatonin levels can impact menstrual cycles.

Interactions and Feedback Mechanisms

The hormonal symphony is not a solo performance; it's a dynamic ensemble where hormones interact and respond to feedback mechanisms to maintain harmony. Let's delve into the intricacies of these interactions and the feedback loops that regulate hormonal balance:

1. **Hypothalamus-Pituitary Axis: The Maestro's Commands:**

- The hypothalamus, a crucial conductor in the endocrine orchestra, releases releasing and inhibiting hormones that signal the pituitary gland. The pituitary gland responds by releasing hormones that stimulate or inhibit other glands, producing specific hormones.

2. Feedback Loop Harmony: Balancing the Score:

- Feedback mechanisms play a pivotal role in hormonal balance. When hormone levels deviate from the desired range, feedback loops activate to increase or decrease hormone production. This ensures that the body maintains homeostasis.

- For example, in regulating thyroid hormones, low levels of thyroid hormone trigger the hypothalamus to release thyrotropin-releasing hormone (TRH), which stimulates the pituitary to release thyroid-stimulating hormone (TSH). TSH then prompts the thyroid gland to produce more thyroid hormones. As thyroid hormone levels rise, they send signals back to the hypothalamus and pituitary, inhibiting further release of TRH and TSH.

3. Negative Feedback: Restoring Equilibrium:

- Negative feedback is a common mechanism where the end product of a process inhibits its production. It acts like a thermostat, maintaining hormonal balance. Elevated levels of a hormone signal the body to decrease production and vice versa.

- For example, insulin helps regulate blood sugar levels. When blood sugar is high, insulin is released to facilitate glucose uptake by cells. As cells take up glucose, blood sugar levels decrease, signaling the pancreas to reduce insulin secretion.

4. Positive Feedback: Amplifying Signals:

- While less common, positive feedback loops amplify signals, leading to an increase in hormone production. This is often seen in processes that require a rapid and decisive response.

- An example is the luteinizing hormone (LH) surge that triggers ovulation in the menstrual cycle. As estrogen levels rise, they eventually reach a threshold that triggers a surge in LH, leading to the release of an egg from the ovary.

5. Cross-Talk Between Hormonal Systems: The Collaborative Crescendo:

- Hormonal systems do not operate in isolation; they often cross-talk and influence each other. For instance, stress hormones (cortisol and adrenaline) can impact reproductive hormones, potentially affecting menstrual cycles.

6. Circadian Rhythms: The Day-Night Duet:

- Hormones follow circadian rhythms, synchronized with the body's internal clock. This influences the timing of hormone release, such as the peak in cortisol levels in the morning to aid wakefulness and the rise in melatonin at night to promote sleep.

CHAPTER 2

Hormonal Imbalances in Women.

The intricate dance of hormones in a woman's body is a finely tuned symphony, and when the notes fall out of harmony, it can manifest as hormonal imbalances. These imbalances can influence various aspects, from the menstrual cycle to mood and overall well-being. Let's explore the terrain of hormonal imbalances in women:

1. Menstrual Irregularities: The Unraveling Cadence:

- Hormonal imbalances often manifest as irregularities in the menstrual cycle. This may include irregular periods, heavy or light bleeding, or even the absence of menstruation (amenorrhea). Fluctuations in estrogen and progesterone levels can disrupt the finely orchestrated sequence of events that govern the menstrual cycle.

2. Polycystic Ovary Syndrome (PCOS): A Dissonant Composition:

- PCOS is characterized by elevated androgen (male hormone) levels, insulin resistance, and the formation of ovarian cysts. This hormonal imbalance can lead to irregular periods, fertility challenges, and symptoms such as acne and hirsutism.

3. Premenstrual Syndrome (PMS): The Prelude to Menstruation:

- Hormonal shifts in the luteal phase of the menstrual cycle can give rise to PMS. Estrogen and progesterone fluctuations may lead to mood swings, irritability, bloating, and breast tenderness.

4. Menopause: The Hormonal Sunset:

- Menopause marks the end of the reproductive years and significantly declines estrogen and progesterone production. Hormonal imbalances during menopause can result in symptoms like hot flashes, mood changes, and changes in bone density.

5. Thyroid Disorders: Metabolic Symphony Disrupted:

- Disorders such as hypothyroidism or hyperthyroidism can disrupt the thyroid's role in regulating metabolism. Symptoms may include fatigue, weight changes, and disturbances in the menstrual cycle.

6. Stress and Cortisol: The Strain on the Strings:

- Chronic stress can lead to imbalances in cortisol, the stress hormone produced by the adrenal glands. Elevated cortisol levels can impact the menstrual cycle, disrupt sleep, and contribute to conditions like adrenal fatigue.

7. Insulin Resistance: The Glucose Waltz:

- Insulin resistance, often associated with conditions like PCOS, can lead to imbalances in blood sugar levels. This can influence hormones in reproductive health and contribute to symptoms like weight gain and irregular periods.

8. Emotional Well-being: The Mood Melody:

- Hormonal imbalances can have a profound impact on mood and emotional well-being. Fluctuations in estrogen and progesterone, especially during menstrual and menopause, may contribute to mood swings, anxiety, or depression.

9. Reproductive Challenges: Fertility Fugue:

- Hormonal imbalances can affect fertility by disrupting ovulation and the overall reproductive process. Conditions like PCOS or irregular menstrual cycles may pose challenges for conception.

10. **Holistic Approaches to Restoration: The Wellness Symphony:**

- Addressing hormonal imbalances often involves a holistic approach. Lifestyle factors, including nutrition, stress management, regular exercise, and adequate sleep, play crucial roles in restoring hormonal balance.

In navigating the hormonal imbalances in women, understanding the nuances of the body's hormonal symphony is vital. Seeking guidance from healthcare professionals, exploring lifestyle interventions, and fostering a mind-body connection contribute to restoring equilibrium in this complex and beautifully orchestrated dance of hormones.

Common Hormonal Issues

The delicate balance of hormones is integral to overall well-being, and disruptions in this balance can give rise to various hormonal issues. Let's explore some common hormonal challenges that individuals may encounter:

1. **Hypothyroidism: The Sluggish Thyroid Sonata:**

- *Overview:* Hypothyroidism occurs when the thyroid gland doesn't produce enough thyroid hormones (T3 and T4).

- *Symptoms:* Fatigue, weight gain, cold intolerance, dry skin, and constipation.

- *Causes:* Autoimmune thyroiditis (Hashimoto's disease), iodine deficiency, or certain medications.

2. Hyperthyroidism: The Accelerated Thyroid Crescendo:

- *Overview:* Hyperthyroidism results from an overactive thyroid gland, producing excessive thyroid hormones.

- *Symptoms:* Weight loss, rapid heartbeat, anxiety, heat intolerance, and tremors.

- *Causes:* Graves' disease, thyroid nodules, or thyroid inflammation.

3. Polycystic Ovary Syndrome (PCOS): The Androgenic Overture:

- *Overview:* PCOS involves an imbalance in sex hormones, with elevated androgen levels.

- *Symptoms:* Irregular periods, ovarian cysts, acne, hirsutism, and fertility challenges.

- *Causes:* Genetic and environmental factors contribute; insulin resistance is often a component.

4. Diabetes: The Glucose Disharmony:

- *Overview:* Diabetes results from problems with insulin production or function, leading to high blood sugar levels.

- *Symptoms:* Increased thirst, frequent urination, fatigue, and blurred vision.

- *Causes:* Type I diabetes (autoimmune) or Type 2 diabetes (insulin resistance).

5. **Adrenal Fatigue: The Stress Response Interlude:**

- *Overview:* Adrenal fatigue is characterized by disruptions in the cortisol response to stress.

- *Symptoms:* Fatigue, difficulty concentrating, insomnia, and irritability.

- *Causes:* Chronic stress, lack of sleep, or prolonged exposure to stressful situations.

6. **Menopause: The Hormonal Sunset Symphony:**

- *Overview:* Menopause marks the end of menstruation, with a decline in estrogen and progesterone.

- *Symptoms:* Hot flashes, mood swings, sleep disturbances, and vaginal dryness.

- *Causes:* Natural aging process leading to decreased ovarian function.

7. **Hormonal Acne: The Dermatological Discord:**

- *Overview:* Hormonal fluctuations in significantly elevated androgen levels can contribute to acne.

- *Symptoms:* Persistent acne, particularly around the jawline and chin.

- *Causes:* Hormonal changes during puberty, menstrual cycle, or conditions like PCOS.

8. **Insulin Resistance: The Glucose Resistance Rhythm:**

- *Overview:* Insulin resistance occurs when cells don't respond well to insulin, leading to elevated blood sugar levels.

- *Symptoms:* Fatigue, increased hunger, and difficulty losing weight.

- *Causes:* Sedentary lifestyle, obesity, genetics, and certain medical conditions.

9. Thyroid Nodules: The Thyroid Nodule Interlude:

- *Overview:* Thyroid nodules are abnormal growths on the thyroid gland.

- *Symptoms:* Often asymptomatic but can cause difficulty swallowing, hoarseness, or neck discomfort.

- *Causes:* Multifactorial, including iodine deficiency or genetic predisposition.

10. Premenstrual Dysphoric Disorder (PMDD): The Menstrual Mood Crescendo:

- *Overview:* PMDD is a severe form of PMS characterized by intense mood disturbances.

- *Symptoms:* Severe mood swings, irritability, and heightened emotional sensitivity.

- *Causes:* The exact cause is unknown; it likely involves hormonal and neurotransmitter fluctuations.

Addressing these hormonal issues often involves a multidimensional approach, incorporating lifestyle modifications, medications, and sometimes hormonal therapy. Seeking guidance from healthcare professionals ensures tailored interventions for optimal hormonal balance.

Polycystic Ovary Syndrome (PCOS)

Polycystic Ovary Syndrome (PCOS) is a multifaceted hormonal disorder that affects individuals assigned to females at birth. This condition involves genetic, hormonal, and environmental factors, leading to various symptoms and potential health implications. Let's delve into the complex landscape of PCOS:

1. Hormonal Imbalance: The Androgenic Overture:

- *Overview:* PCOS is characterized by elevated levels of androgens, often referred to as "male hormones," such as testosterone. This hormonal imbalance can disrupt the typical menstrual cycle and contribute to various symptoms.

2. Ovulatory Dysfunction: The Menstrual Discord:

- *Symptoms:* Common manifestations include irregular menstrual cycles, anovulation (lack of ovulation), and oligomenorrhea (infrequent periods). This can impact fertility.

3. Ovarian Cysts: The Follicular Ensemble:

- *Physical Manifestation:* While the name suggests cysts, these are tiny, fluid-filled sacs in the ovaries. They result from the failure of follicles to mature and release eggs during ovulation.

4. Insulin Resistance: The Metabolic Interlude:

- *Association:* Many individuals with PCOS exhibit insulin resistance, where cells don't respond effectively to insulin. This can lead to elevated insulin levels and increased androgen production.

5. **Symptoms: The Varied Melodies of PCOS:**

- *Common Symptoms:* Alongside menstrual irregularities, PCOS may present with symptoms such as acne, hirsutism (excessive facial or body hair growth), and alopecia (hair loss).

6. **Metabolic Complications: The Glucose Harmony Disrupted:**

- *Association:* Insulin resistance in PCOS can increase the risk of developing metabolic complications, including type 2 diabetes and cardiovascular issues.

7. **Fertility Challenges: The Reproductive Dilemma:**

- *Impact:* Irregular ovulation can result in difficulties conceiving. However, with appropriate management, many individuals with PCOS can achieve successful pregnancies.

8. **Management Strategies: The Treatment Symphony:**

- *Lifestyle Interventions:* Healthy lifestyle choices, including regular exercise, balanced nutrition, and weight management, can help manage symptoms and improve insulin sensitivity.

- *Medications:* Hormonal contraceptives, anti-androgen drugs, and medications to induce ovulation (for fertility concerns) are often prescribed.

- *Management of Metabolic Issues:* Addressing insulin resistance through medications like metformin may be recommended.

9. **Individualized Care: The Personalized Composition:**

- *Approach:* PCOS varies widely among individuals, and treatment plans should be tailored to address specific symptoms and concerns. A collaborative approach with healthcare professionals is crucial.

10. Emotional Well-being: The Mind-Body Symphony:

- *Impact:* PCOS can have emotional and psychological implications. Managing stress, seeking support, and addressing mental health concerns are integral to holistic care.

Navigating PCOS involves understanding its diverse manifestations and adopting a personalized approach to management. With comprehensive care that considers hormonal, metabolic, and emotional aspects, individuals with PCOS can lead fulfilling and healthy lives.

Thyroid Disorders

The thyroid, a small butterfly-shaped gland in the neck, regulates metabolism, energy production, and overall well-being. Thyroid disorders encompass a range of conditions that affect the thyroid's function, leading to various symptoms and health implications. Let's explore the landscape of thyroid disorders:

1. Hypothyroidism: The Sluggish Thyroid Sonata:

- *Overview:* Hypothyroidism occurs when the thyroid gland doesn't produce enough thyroid hormones (T3 and T4).

- *Symptoms:* Fatigue, weight gain, cold intolerance, dry skin, and constipation.

- *Causes:* Autoimmune thyroiditis (Hashimoto's disease), iodine deficiency, or certain medications.

2. Hyperthyroidism: The Accelerated Thyroid Crescendo:

- *Overview:* Hyperthyroidism results from an overactive thyroid gland, producing excessive thyroid hormones.

- *Symptoms:* Weight loss, rapid heartbeat, anxiety, heat intolerance, and tremors.

- *Causes:* Graves' disease, thyroid nodules, or thyroid inflammation.

3. Thyroid Nodules: The Thyroid Nodule Interlude:

- *Overview:* Thyroid nodules are abnormal growths on the thyroid gland.

- *Symptoms:* Often asymptomatic but can cause difficulty swallowing, hoarseness, or neck discomfort.

- *Causes:* Multifactorial, including iodine deficiency or genetic predisposition.

4. Thyroiditis: The Inflammatory Overture:

- *Overview:* Thyroiditis involves inflammation of the thyroid gland, impacting hormone production.

- *Symptoms:* Neck pain, fatigue, and signs of hyperthyroidism or hypothyroidism, depending on the phase.

- *Causes:* Autoimmune (Hashimoto's thyroiditis), viral infections, or medications.

5. Graves 'disease: The Immune Symphony in Hyperdrive:

- *Overview:* Graves' disease is an autoimmune disorder where the immune system attacks the thyroid, leading to hyperthyroidism.

- *Symptoms:* Bulging eyes (exophthalmos), weight loss, anxiety, and rapid heartbeat.

- *Causes:* Autoimmune dysfunction, genetic predisposition.

6. Hashimoto's Disease: The Autoimmune Lament:

- *Overview:* Hashimoto's disease is an autoimmune condition where the immune system targets and damages the thyroid, causing hypothyroidism.

- *Symptoms:* Fatigue, weight gain, depression, and sensitivity to cold.

- *Causes:* Autoimmune dysfunction, genetic factors.

7. Congenital Hypothyroidism: The Newborn Prelude:

- *Overview:* Congenital hypothyroidism occurs from birth, where the thyroid doesn't develop or function properly.

- *Symptoms:* Jaundice, poor feeding, and developmental delays if left untreated.

- *Causes:* Genetic factors or problems with thyroid development in utero.

8. Thyroid Cancer: The Unsettled Melody:

- *Overview:* Thyroid cancer involves the abnormal growth of cells in the thyroid gland.

- *Symptoms:* Lump in the neck, hoarseness, and difficulty swallowing.

- *Causes:* Genetic factors, exposure to radiation, or unknown factors.

9. Thyroid Storm: The Urgent Crescendo:

- *Overview:* Thyroid storm is a rare, life-threatening complication of hyperthyroidism.

- *Symptoms:* Extreme fever, rapid heartbeat, and confusion.

- *Causes:* Often triggered by stress, infection, or uncontrolled hyperthyroidism.

10. Management Strategies: The Treatment Symphony:

- *Medications:* Thyroid hormone replacement for hypothyroidism, anti-thyroid medicines for hyperthyroidism.

- *Radioactive iodine therapy:* Used for hyperthyroidism or certain thyroid cancers.

- *Surgery:* Partial or complete thyroidectomy for specific conditions.

Recognizing Symptoms

Being attuned to the language your body speaks is crucial to maintaining well-being. Here's a guide to recognizing symptoms that might signal underlying health concerns:

1. Fatigue: The Silent Alarm Bell:

- *Potential Causes:* Various factors, including sleep deprivation, stress, anemia, thyroid disorders, or chronic conditions.

- *Red Flags:* Persistent fatigue that doesn't improve with rest, especially if accompanied by other symptoms.

2. Changes in Weight: The Unseen Indicator:

- *Potential Causes:* Thyroid disorders (hypothyroidism or hyperthyroidism), diabetes, hormonal imbalances, or changes in diet and activity.

- *Red Flags:* Unexplained weight loss or gain, especially if rapid or accompanied by other symptoms.

3. Digestive Discomfort: The Gut's Whisper:

- *Potential Causes:* Dietary factors, gastrointestinal issues, stress, or infections.

- *Red Flags:* Persistent digestive symptoms such as bloating, abdominal pain, or changes in bowel habits.

4. Joint Pain: The Body's S.O.S.:

- *Potential Causes:* Inflammatory conditions, arthritis, injuries, or autoimmune disorders.

- *Red Flags:* Persistent or worsening joint pain, especially if accompanied by swelling or stiffness.

5. Changes in Skin: The External Manifestation:

- *Potential Causes:* Allergies, dermatological conditions, hormonal imbalances, or systemic diseases.

- *Red Flags:* New or changing moles, persistent rashes, or unusual skin changes.

6. Mood Changes: The Emotional Barometer:

- *Potential Causes:* Stress, hormonal fluctuations, mental health conditions, or life changes.

- *Red Flags:* Persistent changes in mood, significantly impacting daily functioning or quality of life.

7. Cognitive Changes: The Mind's Whispers:

- *Potential Causes:* Sleep deprivation, stress, neurological conditions, or medication side effects.

- *Red Flags:* Memory loss, confusion, or difficulty concentrating that interferes with daily tasks.

8. **Respiratory Symptoms: The Breath of Concern:**

- *Potential Causes:* Infections, allergies, respiratory conditions, or environmental factors.

- *Red Flags:* Persistent cough, shortness of breath, or chest pain.

9. **Cardiovascular Changes: The Heart's Signals:**

- *Potential Causes:* High blood pressure, heart conditions, or lifestyle factors.

- *Red Flags:* Chest pain, palpitations, or unexplained changes in blood pressure.

10. **Changes in Urination: The Fluid Communication:**

- *Potential Causes:* Dehydration, urinary tract infections, kidney issues, or diabetes.

- *Red Flags:* Frequent urination, pain or discomfort, or changes in urine color.

11. **Reproductive Changes: The Hormonal Notations:**

- *Potential Causes:* Pregnancy, hormonal imbalances, or gynecological conditions.

- *Red Flags:* Changes in menstrual cycle, fertility challenges, or unusual symptoms related to reproductive health.

12. **Vision Changes: The Window to Health:**

- *Potential Causes:* Eye conditions, neurological issues, or systemic diseases.

- *Red Flags:* Blurred vision, double vision, or sudden changes in visual acuity.

13. Fever: The Body's Defense Mechanism:

- *Potential Causes:* Infections, inflammatory conditions, or systemic illnesses.

- *Red Flags:* Persistent or unexplained fever, especially if accompanied by other symptoms.

14. Persistent Pain: The Body's SOS Signal:

- *Potential Causes:* Injuries, chronic conditions, inflammation, or infections.

- *Red Flags:* Unexplained or worsening pain that persists over time.

15. Sleep Disturbances: The Night's Messages:

- *Potential Causes:* Stress, sleep disorders, hormonal imbalances, or lifestyle factors.

- *Red Flags:* Chronic insomnia, excessive sleepiness, or changes in sleep patterns.

Listening to Your Body: The Ongoing Conversation:

- Pay attention to persistent or unusual symptoms.

- Please keep track of changes in your body, including their frequency and intensity.

- Don't hesitate to seek medical advice if you have concerns about your health.

Remember, your body communicates in its unique language, and recognizing the subtle whispers of symptoms allows you to respond proactively to maintain your well-being. Consulting with a healthcare professional is always wise if you have specific questions or concerns about symptoms.

Physical Signs

Our bodies often communicate through physical signs—observable changes that may indicate underlying health considerations. Here's a guide to recognizing and understanding some common physical symptoms:

1. Skin Changes: The External Canvas:

- *Signs:* Changes in color, texture, or the appearance of moles.

- *Possible Causes:* Sun exposure, dermatological conditions, or systemic diseases.

- *Considerations:* Regularly check your skin for new or changing moles. Consult a dermatologist for concerns.

2. Hair and Nail Changes: The Tresses and Cuticles Chronicle:

- *Signs:* Hair loss, texture changes, or nail appearance alterations.

- *Possible Causes:* Hormonal imbalances, nutritional deficiencies, or certain health conditions.

- *Considerations:* Address underlying causes and ensure a balanced diet for healthy hair and nails.

3. Swelling: The Fluid Expression:

- *Signs:* Edema or swelling in various body parts.

- *Possible Causes:* Fluid retention, circulatory issues, or inflammatory conditions.

- *Considerations:* Consult a healthcare professional if the node is persistent or sudden.

4. Changes in Eyes: The Windows to Health:

- *Signs:* Redness, irritation, changes in vision, or bulging eyes.

- *Possible Causes:* Infections, allergies, thyroid disorders, or other eye conditions.

- *Considerations:* Seek an eye examination for persistent or concerning changes.

5. Facial Expression: The Emotional Mirror:

- *Signs:* Changes in facial expression, drooping, or asymmetry.

- *Possible Causes:* Neurological issues, Bell's palsy, or facial nerve disorders.

- *Considerations:* Seek medical attention for sudden changes in facial expression.

6. Posture and Gait: The Movement Memoirs:

- *Signs:* Changes in posture, walking patterns, or balance.

- *Possible Causes:* Musculoskeletal issues, neurological conditions, or injuries.

- *Considerations:* Consult with a healthcare professional for persistent changes in movement.

7. Breathing Patterns: The Respiratory Rhythms:

- *Signs:* Shortness of breath, rapid breathing, or labored breathing.

- *Possible Causes:* Respiratory conditions, cardiovascular issues, or anxiety.

- *Considerations:* Seek medical attention for persistent or severe breathing changes.

8. Changes in Body Weight: The Balance Sheet:

- *Signs:* Unexplained weight loss or gain.

- *Possible Causes:* Thyroid disorders, hormonal imbalances, or underlying health conditions.

- *Considerations:* Consult a healthcare professional for significant and unexplained changes in weight.

9. Muscle Tone and Strength: The Physical Symphony:

- *Signs:* Changes in muscle tone, weakness, or muscle atrophy.

- *Possible Causes:* Neuromuscular disorders, injuries, or systemic diseases.

- *Considerations:* Consult with a healthcare professional for persistent muscle-related concerns.

10. Temperature Changes: The Thermoregulatory Tale:

- *Signs:* Cold extremities, excessive sweating, or intolerance to temperature changes.

- *Possible Causes:* Thyroid disorders, circulatory issues, or hormonal imbalances.

- *Considerations:* Investigate persistent changes in body temperature.

11. Dental and Oral Changes: The Mouth Memo:

- *Signs:* Changes in gum health, mouth sores, or oral discomfort.

- *Possible Causes:* Dental issues, nutritional deficiencies, or systemic conditions.

- *Considerations:* Regular dental check-ups and seeking care for persistent oral changes.

12. Tremors or Shaking: The Vibrato:

- *Signs:* Involuntary tremors or shaking.

- *Possible Causes:* Neurological conditions, anxiety, or medication side effects.

- *Considerations:* Consult a healthcare professional for persistent or concerning tremors.

13. Digestive Changes: The Gastronomic Gazette:

- *Signs:* Changes in bowel habits, abdominal pain, or digestive discomfort.

- *Possible Causes:* Gastrointestinal issues, dietary factors, or inflammatory conditions.

- *Considerations:* Seek medical advice for persistent digestive concerns.

14. Heart Rate and Blood Pressure: The Cardiovascular Codes:

- *Signs:* Changes in heart rate or blood pressure.

- *Possible Causes:* Cardiovascular issues, stress, or hormonal imbalances.

- *Considerations:* Monitor and seek medical attention for significant or persistent changes.

15. **Changes in Breast Tissue: The Mammary Messages:**

- *Signs:* Changes in breast size, lumps, or nipple discharge.

- *Possible Causes:* Hormonal fluctuations, cysts, or breast conditions.

- *Considerations:* Regular breast self-exams and consultation with a healthcare professional for concerns.

Remember:

- A healthcare professional should evaluate changes that persist or worsen.

- Regular health check-ups and screenings are essential for maintaining overall well-being.

- Trust your instincts—if something feels off, seek medical advice.

Attention to physical signs allows for early detection and intervention, contributing to optimal health and well-being.

Emotional and Behavioral Signs

Our emotions and behaviors often serve as windows into our mental well-being. Recognizing and understanding these signs is crucial for maintaining mental health. Here's a guide to emotional and behavioral symptoms that may warrant attention:

1. **Mood Swings: The Emotional Rollercoaster:**

- *Characters:* Rapid shifts in mood, from euphoria to sadness or irritability.

- *Possible Causes:* Hormonal fluctuations, stress, or mental health conditions.

- *Considerations:* Persistent or extreme mood swings may indicate underlying emotional challenges.

2. Changes in Sleep Patterns: The Nighttime Symphony:

- *Signs:* Insomnia, excessive sleepiness, or irregular sleep patterns.

- *Possible Causes:* Stress, anxiety, depression, or sleep disorders.

- *Considerations:* Consistent disturbances in sleep may impact mental well-being.

3. Appetite Changes: The Gastronomic Emotions:

- *Signs:* Significant changes in appetite, either increased or decreased.

- *Possible Causes:* Stress, depression, or eating disorders.

- *Considerations:* Pay attention to persistent changes in eating habits.

4. Social Withdrawal: The Solitary Silence:

- *Signs:* Avoidance of social interactions, isolation, or disengagement.

- *Possible Causes:* Depression, anxiety, or overwhelming stress.

- *Considerations:* Social withdrawal may signal emotional distress.

5. Irritability: The Emotional Edginess:

- *Signs:* Increased sensitivity, impatience, or heightened irritability.

- *Possible Causes:* Stress, hormonal changes, or mood disorders.

- *Considerations:* Excessive irritability may impact relationships and daily functioning.

6. Loss of Interest: The Passion Play:

- *Signs:* Diminished interest or pleasure in activities once enjoyed.

- *Possible Causes:* Depression, burnout, or anhedonia (inability to experience joy).

- *Considerations:* Persistent loss of interest may indicate emotional distress.

7. Difficulty Concentrating: The Cognitive Fog:

- *Signs:* Challenges focusing, forgetfulness, or mental fog.

- *Possible Causes:* Stress, anxiety, depression, or attention disorders.

- *Considerations:* Cognitive difficulties may impact work or academic performance.

8. Changes in Energy Levels: The Vitality Variations:

- *Signs:* Fatigue, low energy, or excessive restlessness.

- *Possible Causes:* Depression, anxiety, or medical conditions affecting energy levels.

- *Considerations:* Significant and persistent changes in energy may reflect emotional struggles.

9. Agitation: The Restless Rhythm:

- *Signs:* Restlessness, pacing, or a sense of inner tension.

- *Possible Causes:* Anxiety, side effects of medications, or neurological conditions.

- *Considerations:* Persistent agitation may indicate emotional unease.

10. Changes in Motivation: The Drive Dilemma:

- *Signs:* Decreased motivation, lack of interest in goal-setting.

- *Possible Causes:* Depression, burnout, or lack of purpose.

- *Considerations:* Assessing and addressing motivation levels is crucial for mental well-being.

11. Emotional Numbness: The Feelings Fading:

- *Signs:* Difficulty experiencing emotions, a sense of emotional numbness.

- *Possible Causes:* Trauma, depression, or dissociation.

- *Considerations:* Emotional numbness may indicate underlying psychological distress.

12. Excessive Worry: The Anxious Anthem:

- *Signs:* Persistent and excessive worry, anticipating the worst outcomes.

- *Possible Causes:* Generalized anxiety disorder, stress, or perfectionism.

- *Considerations:* Chronic worry may impact mental and physical well-being.

13. **Changes in Self-Esteem: The Self-Image Symphony:**

- *Signs:* Fluctuations in self-esteem, negative self-talk, or self-doubt.

- *Possible Causes:* Depression, anxiety, or body image concerns.

- *Considerations:* Monitoring and addressing self-esteem fluctuations is essential.

14. **Excessive Guilt or Shame: The Emotional Burden:**

- *Signs:* Persistent feelings of guilt or shame, self-blame.

- *Possible Causes:* Depression, trauma, or unresolved emotional issues.

- *Considerations:* Excessive guilt may contribute to emotional distress.

15. **Suicidal Thoughts: The Critical Crescendo:**

- *Signs:* Expressing thoughts of suicide, feeling hopeless or overwhelmed.

- *Possible Causes:* Severe depression, anxiety, or other mental health conditions.

- *Considerations:* Suicidal thoughts require immediate professional intervention.

Prioritizing Mental Well-being:

- Regular self-check-ins for emotional well-being are essential.

- Seeking support from friends, family, or mental health professionals is a sign of strength.

- Understanding that mental health is integral to overall well-being.

Recognizing emotional and behavioral signs allows for early intervention and support.

CHAPTER 3

Nourishing Your Body for Hormonal Harmony

In the intricate orchestration of hormonal balance, the role of nutrition cannot be overstated. The foods we choose to nourish our bodies support hormonal harmony, influencing everything from menstrual regularity to mood stability. Here's a note on the significance of raising your body for hormonal well-being:

I. Balancing Macronutrients: The Nutrient Ballet:

- *Proteins:* Essential for hormone synthesis and balance. Include sources like lean meats, poultry, fish, legumes, and plant-based proteins.

- *Healthy Fats:* Omega-3 fatty acids in fatty fish, flaxseeds, and walnuts contribute to hormonal balance and anti-inflammatory effects.

- *Complex Carbohydrates:* Whole grains, fruits, and vegetables provide fiber and help regulate blood sugar levels, impacting insulin and other hormones.

2. Mindful Eating: The Gastronomic Symphony:

- *Slow Eating:* Cultivate a habit of slow, mindful eating. This supports digestion and may positively impact hormones related to satiety and metabolism.

- *Sensory Enjoyment:* Engage your senses while eating. Appreciate your meals' colors, textures, and flavors to enhance the pleasure of nourishment.

Nutrient-Rich Foods for Hormonal Balance

Nourishing your body with nutrient-rich foods is akin to conducting a harmonious symphony within. These foods provide the essential building blocks for hormonal balance, influencing your well-being. Here's a guide to nutrient-rich foods that contribute to hormonal harmony:

1. Fatty Fish: The Omega-3 Overture:

- *Salmon, mackerel, and sardines:* Rich in omega-3 fatty acids, these fish support the production of hormones and have anti-inflammatory properties.

2. Leafy Greens: The Verdant Vibrato:

- *Spinach, kale, and Swiss chard:* Packed with nutrients like vitamin B, magnesium, and antioxidants, leafy greens support overall hormonal health.

3. Avocado: The Creamy Crescendo:

- *Avocado:* A source of monounsaturated fats, avocados provide healthy fats that support hormone production and balance.

4. Berries: The Antioxidant Aria:

- *Blueberries, strawberries, and raspberries:* Rich in antioxidants, berries combat oxidative stress and contribute to overall well-being.

5. Nuts and Seeds: The Nutrient Ensemble:

- *Almonds, walnuts, chia seeds, and flaxseeds:* These are sources of healthy fats, fiber, and essential minerals, supporting hormonal balance.

6. Lean Proteins: The Protein Sonata:

- *Chicken, turkey, tofu, and legumes:* Lean proteins provide amino acids necessary for hormone synthesis and overall cellular function.

7. Whole Grains: The Fiber Refrain:

- *Quinoa, brown rice, and oats:* Whole grains offer fiber, support digestive health, and help regulate blood sugar levels.

8. Broccoli and Cauliflower: The Cruciferous Concerto:

- *Broccoli and cauliflower:* Cruciferous vegetables contain compounds that support liver detoxification, aiding in hormone balance.

9. Greek Yogurt: The Probiotic Prelude:

- *Greek yogurt:* A source of probiotics that promote gut health. A healthy gut is linked to improved hormonal balance.

10. Dark Chocolate: The Cocoa Cadence:

- *Dark chocolate:* In moderation, dark chocolate can be a delightful treat rich in antioxidants and mood-enhancing compounds.

11. Citrus Fruits: The Vitamin C Serenade:

- *Oranges, grapefruits, and lemons:* Citrus fruits provide vitamin C, synthesizing adrenal hormones.

12. Pumpkin Seeds: The Zinc Zephyr:

- *Pumpkin seeds:* A rich source of zinc, crucial for hormonal balance and immune function.

13. Turmeric: The Spice Harmony:

- *Turmeric:* Contains curcumin, known for its anti-inflammatory properties, supporting overall health.

14. Beets: The Nitric Oxide Notes:

- *Beets:* Rich in nitrates, beets support blood flow and cardiovascular health, indirectly impacting hormonal balance.

15. Eggs: The Protein Pianissimo:

- *Eggs:* A complete protein source with essential amino acids, supporting muscle health and hormonal balance.

Remember:

- Variety is vital; aim for a diverse range of nutrient-rich foods.

- Mindful eating promotes better digestion and nutrient absorption.

- Moderation is essential; balance your dietary choices for overall well-being.

Essential Nutrients for Hormones

The intricate dance of hormones within the body relies on a symphony of essential nutrients. These nutrients act as building blocks, supporting hormones' synthesis, regulation, and balance. Here's a spotlight on the vital nutrients crucial for hormonal harmony:

1. **Omega-3 Fatty Acids: The Harmonious Lipids:**

- *Sources:* Fatty fish (salmon, mackerel, sardines), flaxseeds, chia seeds, walnuts.

- *Role:* Omega-3s contribute to the production of anti-inflammatory hormones and support overall hormonal balance.

2. **Vitamin D: The Sunshine Vitamin:**

- *Sources:* Sun exposure, fatty fish, fortified dairy products, eggs.

- *Role:* Vitamin D is essential for synthesizing various hormones, including the active form of vitamin D, which acts as a hormone in the body.

3. **Vitamin B Complex: The Energy Ensemble:**

- *Sources:* Whole grains, lean meats, poultry, fish, eggs, dairy, leafy greens.

- *Role:* B vitamins, including B6, B12, and folate, are crucial in energy production and synthesizing neurotransmitters and hormones.

4. **Zinc: The Hormonal Helper:**

- *Sources:* Pumpkin seeds, chickpeas, lentils, beef, poultry, dairy.

- *Role:* Zinc synthesizes various hormones, including insulin and sex hormones, and supports immune function.

5. **Magnesium: The Relaxation Mineral:**

- *Sources:* Leafy greens, nuts, seeds, whole grains, legumes.

- *Role:* Magnesium regulates cortisol, the stress hormone, and supports muscle and nerve function.

6. Protein: The Amino Acid Anthem:

- *Sources:* Lean meats, poultry, fish, tofu, legumes, dairy.

- *Role:* Amino acids from protein sources are fundamental for synthesizing hormones, enzymes, and neurotransmitters.

7. Vitamin C: The Antioxidant Serenade:

- *Sources:* Citrus fruits, strawberries, bell peppers, broccoli.

- *Role:* Vitamin C supports adrenal gland function and collagen synthesis, which is crucial for skin health and hormone production.

8. Iron: The Oxygen Conductor:

- *Sources:* Red meat, poultry, fish, beans, lentils, fortified cereals.

- *Role:* Iron is essential for oxygen transport in the blood and supports thyroid function.

9. Iodine: The Thyroid Maestro:

- *Sources:* Seafood, iodized salt, dairy products.

- *Role:* Iodine is a crucial component of thyroid hormones, essential for regulating metabolism.

10. Selenium: The Antioxidant Synergy:

- *Sources:* Brazil nuts, seafood, poultry, eggs.

- *Role:* Selenium converts thyroid hormones and acts as an antioxidant.

11. **Fiber: The Digestive Harmony:**

- *Sources:* Whole grains, fruits, vegetables, legumes.

- *Role:* Dietary fiber supports gut health, aiding in the elimination of excess hormones and promoting hormonal balance.

12. **Probiotics: The Gut Guardians:**

- *Sources:* Yogurt, kefir, sauerkraut, kimchi.

- *Role:* Probiotics contribute to gut health, influencing the metabolism and balance of hormones.

13. **Choline: The Brain and Hormone Liaison:**

- *Sources:* Eggs, liver, salmon, peanuts.

- *Role:* Choline is involved in neurotransmitter synthesis and supports hormonal balance, especially during pregnancy.

14. **Vitamin E: The Antioxidant Ensemble:**

- *Sources:* Nuts, seeds, spinach, broccoli, sunflower oil.

- *Role:* Vitamin E is an antioxidant, supporting overall cell health and hormonal balance.

15. **Phytoestrogens: The Plant Harmony:**

- *Sources:* Soy products, flaxseeds, lentils, chickpeas.

- *Role:* Phytoestrogens, plant compounds with estrogen-like properties, can modulate hormone activity in the body.

Remember:

- A balanced and varied diet provides a spectrum of essential nutrients.

- Nutrient needs may vary based on individual factors, including age, gender, and health status.

- Consult with a healthcare professional or a registered dietitian for personalized nutritional guidance.

Foods to Support Hormone Production

Nourishing your body with foods that support hormone production is a proactive approach to maintaining overall well-being. These nutrient-rich foods provide the building blocks and cofactors necessary for synthesizing and regulating hormones. Here's a selection of foods that play a key role in supporting hormonal harmony:

1. Salmon: The Omega-3 Maestro:

- *Omega-3 Fatty Acids:* Essential for hormone production, omega-3s in salmon support synthesizing prostaglandins and anti-inflammatory hormones.

2. Eggs: The Protein Pinnacle:

- *Protein and Choline:* Eggs are rich in protein, providing amino acids crucial for hormone synthesis. Choline supports liver function, aiding in hormone metabolism.

3. Avocado: The Monounsaturated Marvel:

- *Healthy Fats:* Avocados contain monounsaturated fats that support the production of cholesterol, a precursor to steroid hormones.

4. Brazil Nuts: The Selenium Sentinel:

- *Selenium:* Brazil nuts are a potent source of selenium, a mineral essential for thyroid hormone synthesis and function.

5. Lean Meats: The Protein Prodigy:

- *Protein and Iron:* Lean meats provide high-quality protein and iron, essential for synthesizing various hormones, including hemoglobin and thyroid hormones.

6. Greek Yogurt: The Probiotic Powerhouse:

- *Probiotics and Protein:* Greek yogurt offers probiotics for gut health and provides the protein necessary for hormonal balance.

7. Berries: The Antioxidant Ensemble:

- *Antioxidants:* Berries are rich in antioxidants that combat oxidative stress, supporting overall cell health and hormonal balance.

8. Broccoli: The Cruciferous Conductor:

- *Indole-3-Carbinol:* Broccoli and other cruciferous vegetables contain compounds like indole-3-carbinol that may support estrogen metabolism.

9. Pumpkin Seeds: The Zinc Zenith:

- *Zinc:* Pumpkin seeds are a valuable zinc source for synthesizing sex hormones and insulin.

10. Oats: The Fiber Forte:

- *Fiber:* Oats provide fiber that aids in digestion and helps regulate blood sugar levels, indirectly impacting hormone balance.

11. **Tofu: The Soy Serenade:**

- *Phytoestrogens:* Tofu and other soy products contain phytoestrogens, plant compounds that may modulate estrogen activity in the body.

12. **Dark Leafy Greens: The Nutrient Nexus:**

- *Vitamins and Minerals:* Greens like spinach and kale provide changes in vitamins and minerals, supporting overall hormonal health.

13. **Quinoa: The Protein Powerhouse:**

- *Complete Protein:* Quinoa is a whole protein source, supplying all essential amino acids for hormone synthesis.

14. **Almonds: The Magnesium Marvel:**

- *Magnesium:* Almonds are a rich source of magnesium, a mineral essential for regulating cortisol and other hormones.

15. **Flaxseeds: The Omega-3 Overture:**

- *Omega-3 Fatty Acids:* Flaxseeds offer a plant-based source of omega-3s, supporting hormone production and anti-inflammatory responses.

16. **Bell Peppers: The Vitamin C Crescendo:**

- *Vitamin C:* Bell peppers provide vitamin C, essential for adrenal gland function and collagen synthesis.

17. **Turmeric: The Curcumin Concerto:**

- *Curcumin:* Turmeric contains curcumin, known for its anti-inflammatory properties and potential to support hormonal balance.

18. **Lentils: The Protein Pulse:**

- *Protein and Fiber:* Lentils combine protein and fiber, supporting digestive health and hormone regulation.

Remember:

- **Diversity is Key:** A varied and balanced diet ensures a broad spectrum of nutrients for hormonal health.

- **Whole Foods Matter:** Opt for whole, unprocessed foods to maximize nutrient intake.

- **Mindful Eating:** Pay attention to hunger and fullness cues, fostering a healthy relationship with food.

The Role of Hydration in Wellness

Water, the elixir of life, is pivotal in maintaining overall wellness. Hydration is not merely a physiological need; it's a cornerstone of vitality that influences every aspect of well-being. Here's a deep dive into the multifaceted role of hydration in supporting your journey to optimal health:

1. Cellular Function: The Aquatic Essence:

- *Transport of Nutrients:* Water is the medium through which nutrients are transported to cells, facilitating essential processes like nutrient absorption and waste removal.

- *Cellular Metabolism:* Adequate hydration is crucial for efficient cellular metabolism, supporting the production of energy and the synthesis of biomolecules.

2. Temperature Regulation: The Coolant Symphony:

- *Thermoregulation:* Sweating is the body's natural cooling mechanism. Proper hydration helps regulate body temperature, preventing overheating during physical activity or in hot environments.

- *Electrolyte Balance:* Hydration maintains the balance of electrolytes, such as sodium and potassium, crucial for nerve function and muscle contractions.

3. Cognitive Function: The Fluid Intelligence:

- *Brain Function:* Water is essential for cognitive processes, including concentration, alertness, and memory. Dehydration can impair cognitive function and lead to difficulties in decision-making.

- *Electrolyte Balance:* Electrolytes, maintained through hydration, support the transmission of nerve signals, influencing cognitive functions and mental clarity.

4. Digestive Health: The Hydrated Digestion:

- *Digestive Enzymes:* Water aids in producing digestive enzymes, supporting the breakdown and absorption of nutrients in the digestive system.

- *Prevention of Constipation:* Adequate hydration softens stool and promotes regular bowel movements, preventing constipation and supporting gut health.

5. Joint Lubrication: The Fluid Cushion:

- *Synovial Fluid:* Hydration is crucial for producing synovial fluid, which lubricates joints and facilitates smooth movement. Dehydration can contribute to joint stiffness and discomfort.

6. Skin Health: The Hydrated Glow:

- *Collagen Production:* Water is essential for synthesizing collagen, a protein that maintains skin elasticity and hydration. Proper hydration contributes to a vibrant and youthful complexion.

- *Toxin Elimination:* Hydration supports the elimination of toxins through sweat and urine, contributing to clearer skin and reducing the risk of skin issues.

7. Detoxification: The Cleansing Cascade:

- *Kidney Function:* Water is vital for kidney function, aiding in the filtration and elimination of waste products from the body. Adequate hydration supports optimal detoxification.

- *Liver Support:* Hydration supports liver function, a key player in detoxification processes. Water helps flush out toxins and metabolic byproducts.

8. Weight Management: The Satiety Symphony:

- *Appetite Regulation:* Drinking water before meals can contribute to a sense of fullness, potentially reducing overall calorie intake and supporting weight management.

- *Metabolic Rate:* Adequate hydration is linked to a healthy metabolic rate, influencing the body's ability to burn calories and maintain a healthy weight.

9. Mood and Energy: The Hydrated Harmony:

- *Fatigue Prevention:* Dehydration can lead to feelings of fatigue and low energy. Staying hydrated supports optimal energy levels throughout the day.

- *Mood Stability:* Hydration plays a role in maintaining mood stability. Even mild dehydration can impact mood and contribute to feelings of irritability.

10. Exercise Performance: The Fluid Endurance:

- *Fluid Balance:* Adequate hydration is crucial for endurance and performance during physical activity. Dehydration can lead to muscle cramps, fatigue, and reduced exercise capacity.

- *Electrolyte Support:* Hydration with electrolyte-rich fluids is essential for replenishing salts lost through sweat during intense exercise.

Practical Tips for Optimal Hydration:

- **Listen to Your Body:** Thirst is a natural indicator of hydration needs. Pay attention to your body's signals.

- **Routine Hydration:** Incorporate regular sips of water throughout the day rather than relying on large amounts at once.

- **Variety in Fluid Intake:** Besides water, include hydrating beverages like herbal teas, infused water, and broths in your routine.

- **Hydration and Nutrition:** Many fruits and vegetables have high water content, contributing to hydration and nutrient intake.

- **Environmental Considerations:** Adjust your fluid intake based on temperature, humidity, and physical activity levels.

- **Personalized Needs:** Individual hydration needs vary based on age, weight, health status, and lifestyle. Consult with healthcare professionals for customized guidance.

<h1 style="text-align:center">Importance of Water in Hormonal Regulation</h1>

Water, often regarded as life's essence, goes beyond quenching thirst—it's a silent conductor in the intricate symphony of hormonal regulation. Its importance extends to every hormonal cue, ensuring the smooth functioning of the endocrine system. Let's delve into the profound significance of water in maintaining hormonal balance:

1. Transportation of Hormones: The Aquatic Pathway:

- *Water as a Medium:* Hormones travel through the bloodstream, and water is the fluid medium for this journey. Proper hydration ensures the efficient transport of hormones to their target tissues, facilitating communication between glands and organs.

2. Synthesis of Hormones: The Hydro-Molecular Dance:

- *Biological Reactions:* The synthesis of hormones often involves complex biochemical reactions. Water is critical in these reactions, providing the aqueous environment for forming hormone molecules.

- *Endocrine Gland Function:* Adequate hydration supports the optimal function of endocrine glands, such as the pituitary, thyroid, and adrenal glands. These glands play key roles in hormone production and regulation.

3. Hormonal Signaling: The Fluid Language:

- *Cellular Communication:* Hormones transmit signals to cells, influencing various physiological processes. Proper hydration ensures these signaling pathways operate smoothly, allowing cells to respond appropriately to hormonal cues.

- *Fluidity of Signaling:* Water enhances the fluidity of intracellular and extracellular environments, facilitating the binding of hormones to receptors and the subsequent transmission of signals.

4. Temperature Regulation: The Hormonal Thermostat:

- *Thyroid Function:* The thyroid gland, a crucial player in hormonal regulation, is sensitive to changes in body temperature. Adequate hydration supports temperature regulation, indirectly influencing thyroid hormone activity.

- *Adrenal Hormones:* Water assists in temperature regulation during physical activities and stress, helping maintain the balance of adrenal hormones, including cortisol.

5. Detoxification: The Cleansing Cascade:

- *Liver Function:* The liver, a central organ in detoxification, relies on water to efficiently process and eliminate toxins. Hydration supports liver health, indirectly influencing hormonal balance.

- *Kidney Filtration:* Proper hydration is essential for kidney function, ensuring the filtration and removal of waste products and excess hormones from the body.

6. Metabolism Support: The Fluid Metabolic Dance:

- *Metabolic Processes:* Water is involved in various metabolic processes, including the breakdown of nutrients for energy. A well-hydrated body supports the metabolic pathways that contribute to hormonal balance.

- *Blood Sugar Regulation:* Hydration influences blood viscosity and circulation, impacting insulin sensitivity and blood sugar regulation.

7. Stress Response: The Calming Hydration:

- *Cortisol Regulation:* Chronic stress can disrupt hormonal balance, particularly cortisol levels. Hydration supports stress resilience, influencing the body's ability to manage cortisol release during stressful situations.

- *Electrolyte Balance:* Water, along with electrolytes, helps maintain the balance of ions in cells, contributing to a stable internal environment during stress responses.

8. Reproductive Hormones: The Fluid Fertility:

- *Menstrual Health:* Proper hydration supports menstrual regularity and hormonal balance in women. Dehydration can impact the menstrual cycle and fertility.

- *Sperm Health:* In men, hydration is linked to sperm health. Maintaining fluid balance supports the production and function of reproductive hormones.

Practical Tips for Hydration and Hormonal Balance:

- **Consistent Hydration:** Maintain a regular water intake pattern throughout the day to support hormonal function.

- **Hydrating Foods:** Include water-rich foods like fruits and vegetables to complement fluid intake.

- **Individual Needs:** Hydration needs vary based on age, weight, physical activity, and climate. Listen to your body's cues for optimal hydration.

- **Caffeine Awareness:** Be mindful of the potential diuretic effect of caffeinated beverages and balance them with water intake.

- **Alcohol Moderation:** If consuming alcohol, balance it with water to prevent dehydration, which can impact hormonal regulation.

- **Regular Monitoring:** Pay attention to signs of dehydration, such as dark urine or increased thirst, and adjust your fluid intake accordingly.

Hydrating Foods and Beverages

Hydration goes beyond just sipping water—it's also about embracing various hydrating foods and beverages that contribute to your body's fluid balance. Here's a curated list of hydrating options that not only quench your thirst but also provide a refreshing and nutritious boost to your overall well-being:

Hydrating Foods: The Nutrient-Rich Quenchers

1. **Cucumber (Water Content: 95%):**

   - *Refreshing Crunch:* Enjoy cucumber slices as a hydrating snack, or add them to salads for a crisp texture and hydration boost.

2. **Watermelon (Water Content: 92%):**

   - *Summertime Favorite:* Watermelon not only hydrates but also provides vitamins and antioxidants. Perfect for a refreshing snack or hydrating smoothies.

3. **Celery (Water Content: 95%):**

   - *Crunchy Stalks:* Celery is not just a low-calorie snack but also a hydrating one. Dip celery sticks in hummus for a satisfying treat.

4. **Strawberries (Water Content: 91%):**

- *Sweet and Juicy:* Strawberries are a delightful source of hydration and vitamin C. Add them to yogurt smoothies, or enjoy them on their own.

5. **Oranges (Water Content: 87%):**

- *Citrus Burst:* Oranges are juicy and rich in vitamin C. Slice them for a hydrating and tangy snack.

6. **Pineapple (Water Content: 86%):**

- *Tropical Twist:* Pineapple adds a sweet and low touch to your hydration routine. Enjoy it fresh, or blend it into a hydrating smoothie.

7. **Bell Peppers (Water Content: 92%):**

- *Colorful Crunch:* Bell peppers, especially the colorful varieties, provide hydration and a burst of vitamins. Dip them in hummus for a satisfying snack.

8. **Lettuce (Iceberg, Water Content: 95%):**

- *Crisp Greens:* Iceberg lettuce is crisp and high in water content. Use it as a base for salads or sandwiches.

9. **Zucchini (Water Content: 95%):**

- *Versatile Veggie:* Zucchini is a hydrating and versatile vegetable. Spiralize it for a hydrating alternative to pasta, or add it to stir-fries.

10. **Tomatoes (Water Content: 94%):**

- *Juicy Delight:* Tomatoes are not only hydrating but also rich in antioxidants. Please include them in salads, sandwiches, or as a sauce base.

Hydrating Beverages: Sip Your Way to Wellness

1. **Water with Lemon:**

   - *Citrus Infusion:* Add a slice of lemon to your water for flavor and vitamin C. It's a simple way to make hydration more enjoyable.

2. **Coconut Water:**

   - *Tropical Hydration:* Coconut water is refreshing and rich in electrolytes, making it a tremendous hydrating beverage, especially after exercise.

3. **Herbal Teas:**

   - *Flavorful Hydration:* Herbal teas, such as peppermint or chamomile, are hydrating alternatives to plain water and offer a variety of flavors.

4. **Infused Water:**

   - *Flavor Fusion:* Infuse water with slices of fruits, vegetables, or herbs for a hydrating beverage with a hint of natural flavor.

5. **Cucumber Mint Cooler:**

   - *Cooling Elixir:* Combine cucumber slices and fresh mint leaves with water for a refreshing and hydrating cooler.

6. **Iced Green Tea:**

- *Antioxidant Boost:* Iced green tea is hydrating and provides antioxidants. Skip or limit added sweeteners for a healthier option.

7. **Watermelon Smoothie:**

   - *Summery Bliss:* Blend watermelon with ice for a hydrating and delicious smoothie. You can also add other hydrating fruits for variety.

8. **Lemonade (with minimal added sugar):**

   - *Classic Refresher:* Freshly squeezed lemonade, with minimal added sugar, is a timeless and hydrating beverage.

9. **Sparkling Water:**

   - *Fizz and Hydration:* Sparkling water, whether plain or flavored, is a bubbly and hydrating alternative to still water.

10. **Homemade Electrolyte Drink:**

    - *DIY Hydration:* Mix water with a pinch of salt and a splash of citrus juice for a homemade electrolyte drink, perfect for replenishing after physical activity.

Tips for Hydrating Success:

- **Set Reminders:** Use reminders or apps to prompt you to drink water regularly throughout the day.

- **Hydrate Before Meals:** Drink water before meals to stay hydrated and potentially support weight management.

- **Carry a Reusable Bottle:** Keep a reusable water bottle with you to make it convenient to sip throughout the day.

- **Listen to Thirst Cues:** Listen to your body's signals and drink when thirsty.

CHAPTER 4

Fasting and Hormonal Brilliance

Embarking on a fasting journey is not merely a break from the eating routine; it's a profound exploration into the intricate dance of hormones that govern your well-being. Fasting, when approached mindfully and with consideration for your body's needs, can act as a catalyst for hormonal brilliance. Let's unravel the symphony between fasting and hormonal harmony:

1. Insulin Sensitivity: The Glucose Maestro:

- *Fasting's Influence:* Intermittent fasting, mainly, has been linked to improved insulin sensitivity. Giving your body periods without constant food intake allows it to regulate blood sugar levels more effectively.

- *Impact on Hormones:* Fasting periods can reduce insulin levels, prompting the body to use stored glucose for energy. This supports metabolic health and influences the balance of other hormones.

2. Growth Hormone Production: The Cellular Conductor:

- *Fasting's Influence:* Short-term fasting has been associated with increased growth hormone levels. Growth hormone is crucial in cellular repair, metabolism, and overall growth.

- *Impact on Hormones:* Elevated growth hormone levels during fasting periods support fat metabolism and muscle preservation and may contribute to overall hormonal balance.

3. Cortisol Regulation: The Stress Symphony:

- *Fasting's Influence:* Intermittent fasting, when done with a balanced approach, may help regulate cortisol levels. Controlled stress on the body during fasting can contribute to resilience and adaptation.

- *Impact on Hormones:* Balanced cortisol levels are crucial for managing stress and maintaining hormonal equilibrium. Fasting, when not overly stressful, can be a part of a holistic approach to cortisol regulation.

4. Leptin and Ghrelin Harmony: The Appetite Duo:

- *Fasting's Influence:* Intermittent fasting patterns can influence the balance between leptin (the satiety hormone) and ghrelin (the hunger hormone). Fasting may contribute to improved appetite regulation.

- *Impact on Hormones:* Achieving a balance in leptin and ghrelin levels supports healthier eating patterns and may contribute to weight management and hormonal stability.

5. Thyroid Function: The Metabolic Orchestra:

- *Fasting's Influence:* Short-term fasting has been studied for its potential impact on thyroid function. Evidence suggests intermittent fasting may influence thyroid hormones without causing long-term harm.

- *Impact on Hormones:* Balancing the delicate interplay of thyroid hormones is crucial for maintaining metabolic health. Fasting, when approached sensibly, may contribute positively to this balance.

6. Autophagy: The Cellular Cleanup Symphony:

- *Fasting's Influence:* Fasting, exceptionally prolonged or intermittent fasting, can stimulate autophagy—an essential cellular process where the body cleans out damaged cells and regenerates new, healthy ones.

- *Impact on Hormones:* Autophagy supports cellular health and longevity, influencing many hormonal processes that contribute to overall well-being.

Tips for Fasting and Hormonal Brilliance:

- **Start Gradually:** If new to fasting, begin with shorter fasting windows and gradually extend them based on your comfort and body's response.

- **Stay Hydrated:** Adequate hydration is essential during fasting periods. Water, herbal teas, and other non-caloric beverages can be included.

- **Mindful Nutrition:** When breaking a fast, focus on nutrient-dense, balanced meals to support hormonal health and provide essential nutrients.

- **Listen to Your Body:** How your body responds to fasting. If you experience significant discomfort or adverse effects, consider adjusting your approach or consulting with a healthcare professional.

- **Variety in Fasting Approaches:** Explore different fasting methods, such as time-restricted eating or intermittent fasting, to find what aligns best with your lifestyle and health goals.

Intermittent Fasting

Intermittent fasting, a time-honored practice with roots in various cultures and traditions, has taken center stage as a contemporary approach to health and wellness. Beyond a dietary trend, intermittent fasting is a rhythmic cycle of eating and fasting, orchestrating a symphony of physiological benefits that resonate throughout the body. Let's explore the critical movements of this intermittent fasting composition:

I. Time-Restricted Eating: The Daily Harmony:

- *The Rhythm:* Time-restricted eating, a popular form of intermittent fasting, involves confining your daily food intake to a specific window. Common patterns include a 16-hour fast with an 8-hour eating window.

- *Metabolic Flexibility:* This approach encourages the body to switch between fed and fasted states, promoting metabolic flexibility. During fasting, the body taps into stored energy, enhancing fat utilization.

2. Autophagy: Cellular Cleanup Overture:

- *The Symphony of Autophagy:* Intermittent fasting stimulates autophagy—a cellular process where the body eliminates damaged or malfunctioning cells. This renewal process contributes to cellular health and longevity.

- *Cellular Detoxification:* Autophagy is akin to a cellular detox, clearing out cellular debris and promoting the regeneration of new, vibrant cells.

3. Insulin Sensitivity: The Glucose Sonata:

- *Balancing Blood Sugar:* Intermittent fasting has been linked to improved insulin sensitivity. With reduced frequency of meals, the body becomes more efficient in managing blood sugar levels.

- *Metabolic Harmony:* Enhanced insulin sensitivity supports metabolic health and may contribute to weight management by optimizing how the body utilizes carbohydrates.

4. Hormonal Modulation: The Endocrine Crescendo:

- *Growth Hormone Symphony:* Intermittent fasting has been associated with increased growth hormone secretion, fostering cellular repair, muscle preservation, and metabolic balance.

- *Leptin and Ghrelin Ballet:* The fasting rhythm influences the balance of appetite-regulating hormones—leptin and ghrelin—promoting a more harmonious relationship with hunger and satiety.

5. Brain Health: The Cognitive Concerto:

- *Neuroprotective Harmony:* Intermittent fasting exhibits neuroprotective effects, supporting brain health and potentially reducing the risk of neurodegenerative conditions.

- *BDNF Melody:* Fasting has been linked to increased levels of brain-derived neurotrophic factor (BDNF), a protein that supports the growth and maintenance of neurons.

6. Inflammation Reduction: The Calming Serenade:

- *Inflammatory Symphony:* Intermittent fasting may contribute to a reduction in systemic inflammation. Lowering inflammation levels is associated with a lower risk of chronic diseases.

- *Oxidative Stress Minuet:* By modulating cellular processes, intermittent fasting may help reduce oxidative stress, contributing to overall cellular health.

Practical Tips for Intermittent Fasting Harmony:

- **Start Gradually:** If new to intermittent fasting, begin with a conservative fasting window and gradually extend it based on your comfort.

- **Hydration is Key:** Stay well-hydrated with water, herbal teas, or other non-caloric beverages during fasting periods.

- **Balanced Nutrition:** Focus on nutrient-dense, balanced meals during eating windows to support overall health and well-being.

- **Listen to Your Body:** Pay attention to your body's signals. If you experience adverse effects, consider adjusting your fasting approach or consulting with a healthcare professional.

- **Variety in Approaches:** Explore different intermittent fasting methods to find what aligns best with your lifestyle and health goals.

Different Approaches to Intermittent Fasting

Intermittent fasting is a flexible and adaptable practice that allows individuals to choose a rhythm that aligns with their lifestyle and health goals. The spectrum of periodic fasting approaches offers diverse options, from daily time-restricted eating to more extended fasting periods. Let's delve into some of the most popular methods:

I. **Time-Restricted Eating (16/8 Method): The Daily Tempo:**

- *The Rhythm:* This method involves a daily fasting window, typically 16 hours, followed by an 8-hour eating window. For example, one might eat between noon and 8 p.m. and fast from 8 p.m. to noon the next day.

- *Flexibility:* It's a practical approach that fits well into daily routines, allowing individuals to choose the timing that suits their lifestyle.

2. Alternate-Day Fasting: The Every Other Day Waltz:

- *The Rhythm:* In alternate-day fasting, individuals alternate between days of regular eating and days of significant calorie restriction or complete fasting.

- *Adaptability:* While some may find this approach challenging, it offers flexibility by allowing normal eating every other day.

3. 5:2 Diet: The Weekly Harmony:

- *The Rhythm:* This method involves regular eating five days a week and two non-consecutive days of significant calorie restriction (usually around 500-600 calories).

- *Sustainability:* The 5:2 diet balances fasting and regular eating, making it more sustainable for some individuals.

4. Eat-Stop-Eat: The Periodic Pause:

- *The Rhythm:* Individuals incorporate one or two 24-hour fasts per week in this approach. For example, eating dinner and not eating until the next day.

- *Variability:* The periodic nature of longer fasts offers a break from routine and can be adapted based on personal preferences.

5. Warrior Diet: The Feasting and Fasting Symphony:

- *The Rhythm:* The Warrior Diet involves eating small amounts of raw fruits and vegetables during the day and having one large meal at night within a 4-hour eating window.

- *Circadian Rhythm:* This method aligns with the body's natural circadian rhythm, emphasizing fasting during the day and feasting in the evening.

6. Extended Fasting (24 Hours or More): The Prolonged Cadence:

- *The Rhythm:* Extended fasting involves fasting for 24 hours or more. Some individuals opt for 36, 48, or even 72-hour fasting periods.

- *Autophagy Boost:* Prolonged fasting may stimulate autophagy more profoundly, offering potential benefits for cellular health and rejuvenation.

7. Spontaneous Meal Skipping: The Impromptu Sonata:

- *The Rhythm:* Some individuals practice intermittent fasting by spontaneously skipping meals when not hungry or based on their daily activities.

- *Flexibility:* This approach is intuitive and flexible, allowing individuals to listen to their body's hunger cues and adjust their eating patterns accordingly.

Tips for Exploring Intermittent Fasting:

- **Personalized Approach:** Choose an intermittent fasting method that aligns with your lifestyle, preferences, and health goals.

- **Start Gradually:** If new to intermittent fasting, begin with a manageable method and gradually experiment with more extended fasting periods if desired.

- **Stay Hydrated:** Drink water, herbal teas, or other non-caloric beverages during fasting periods to stay hydrated.

- **Nutrient-Dense Eating:** When breaking a fast, focus on nutrient-dense, balanced meals to support overall health and well-being.

- **Listen to Your Body:** Pay attention to how your body responds to different fasting methods, and be open to adjusting your approach based on your experiences.

Benefits and Risks of Intermittent Fasting

Intermittent fasting, a practice with roots in various cultures and traditions, has gained popularity for its potential health benefits. While it can offer a range of advantages, it's essential to approach intermittent fasting with an understanding of its benefits and potential risks.

Benefits of Intermittent Fasting:

1. **Metabolic Health Improvement:**

    - *Insulin Sensitivity:* Intermittent fasting may enhance insulin sensitivity, contributing to better blood sugar regulation and a reduced risk of type 2 diabetes.

    - *Weight Management:* By promoting fat utilization during fasting periods, intermittent fasting may support weight management and loss.

2. **Cellular Repair and Longevity:**

- *Autophagy Activation:* Intermittent fasting stimulates autophagy, a process where the body cleans out damaged cells and regenerates new, healthy ones, potentially contributing to longevity.

- *Cellular Detoxification:* The periodic fasting and feasting cycle may act as a form of cellular detoxification, promoting overall cellular health.

3. **Hormonal Balance:**

- *Growth Hormone Release:* Intermittent fasting has been associated with increased secretion of growth hormone, which supports muscle preservation, fat metabolism, and overall hormonal balance.

- *Appetite Regulation:* Balancing appetite-regulating hormones like leptin and ghrelin may contribute to healthier eating patterns and weight management.

4. **Brain Health Enhancement:**

- *Neuroprotective Effects:* Intermittent fasting exhibits neuroprotective effects, potentially reducing the risk of neurodegenerative conditions.

- *Cognitive Function:* The practice may support cognitive function and brain health by promoting the release of brain-derived neurotrophic factor (BDNF), a protein crucial for neuronal growth.

5. **Inflammation Reduction:**

- *Reduced Systemic Inflammation:* Intermittent fasting may contribute to lower levels of systemic inflammation, reducing the risk of chronic diseases associated with inflammation.

6. **Heart Health Benefits:**

- *Blood Lipid Profile:* Some studies suggest that intermittent fasting may improve blood lipid profiles, including cholesterol levels, supporting cardiovascular health.

- *Blood Pressure Regulation:* Intermittent fasting may improve blood pressure regulation, promoting heart health.

Considerations and Risks:

1. **Nutrient Deficiency Risk:**

- *Inadequate Nutrient Intake:* If not approached with balanced nutrition, intermittent fasting may increase the risk of nutrient deficiencies. Ensuring nutrient-dense meals during eating windows is crucial.

2. **Eating Disorders and Disordered Eating:**

- *Potential Triggers:* Intermittent fasting may be a trigger for individuals susceptible to or recovering from eating disorders. It's essential to approach it mindfully and seek professional guidance if needed.

3. **Individual Variability:**

- *Not One-Size-Fits-All:* Intermittent fasting may not be suitable for everyone. Individual responses vary, and some individuals may experience adverse effects, including fatigue, irritability, or disruptions to menstrual cycles.

4. **Potential Stress Response:**

   - *Cortisol Levels:* Prolonged or intense intermittent fasting may lead to elevated cortisol levels, impacting stress response. Balancing fasting with adequate rest and recovery is crucial.

5. **Social and Lifestyle Considerations:**

   - *Social Impact:* Intermittent fasting may pose challenges in social settings where meals are typically shared. It's essential to consider how fasting aligns with personal and social aspects of life.

6. **Medication Interactions:**

   - *Consultation with Healthcare Providers:* Individuals taking medications or with pre-existing health conditions should consult with them before starting intermittent fasting, as it may interact with certain medicines or conditions.

Practical Tips for Safe Intermittent Fasting:

- **Start Gradually:** Begin with shorter fasting periods and gradually increase duration based on comfort and experience.

- **Prioritize Nutrient-Dense Foods:** Ensure meals during eating windows are rich in essential nutrients to prevent deficiencies.

- **Stay Hydrated:** Drink water, herbal teas, or other non-caloric beverages to stay hydrated during fasting periods.

- **Listen to Your Body:** Pay attention to how your body responds to intermittent fasting, and be open to adjusting your approach based on feedback.

- **Professional Guidance:** Consult with healthcare professionals or registered dietitians, especially if you have pre-existing health conditions or concerns.

Intermittent fasting can be a powerful tool for some individuals when approached mindfully and with consideration for individual needs. Balancing its potential benefits with awareness of possible risks ensures a safe and sustainable practice. As you embark on your intermittent fasting journey, may it be guided by wisdom and a commitment to holistic well-being.

Fasting and Hormonal Regulation

Fasting, a practice deeply rooted in human history, has profound effects on hormonal regulation, orchestrating a delicate balance within the intricate symphony of the endocrine system. As you embark on a fasting journey, let's explore the profound interactions between fasting and hormonal dynamics:

I. Insulin Sensitivity: The Glucose Maestro:

- *Fasting's Influence:* During fasting, especially in periods of reduced carbohydrate intake, insulin levels decrease. This prompts the body to use stored glucose for energy, enhancing insulin sensitivity.

- *Impact on Hormones:* Improved insulin sensitivity supports stable blood sugar levels and may reduce the risk of insulin resistance, a precursor to type 2 diabetes.

2. **Growth Hormone Production: The Cellular Conductor:**

- *Fasting's Influence:* Short-term fasting has been associated with increased growth hormone production. Growth hormone is pivotal in cellular repair, metabolism, and preserving lean muscle mass.

- *Impact on Hormones:* Elevated growth hormone levels during fasting contribute to using stored fat for energy, supporting fat loss and overall metabolic health.

3. **Cortisol Regulation: The Stress Symphony:**

- *Fasting's Influence:* Intermittent fasting, when approached with balance, may positively impact cortisol regulation. Controlled stress on the body during fasting can contribute to resilience and adaptation.

- *Impact on Hormones:* A balanced cortisol response supports the body's ability to manage stress and promotes hormonal equilibrium.

4. **Leptin and Ghrelin Harmony: The Appetite Duo:**

- *Fasting's Influence:* Intermittent fasting patterns can modulate the balance between leptin (satiety hormone) and ghrelin (hunger hormone). This may contribute to improved appetite regulation.

- *Impact on Hormones:* Achieving a harmonious balance in leptin and ghrelin levels promotes healthier eating patterns and may aid in weight management.

5. **Thyroid Function: The Metabolic Orchestra:**

- *Fasting's Influence:* Short-term intermittent fasting has been studied for its potential impact on thyroid function. Some evidence suggests that it may influence thyroid hormones without causing long-term harm.

- *Impact on Hormones:* Balancing the delicate interplay of thyroid hormones is crucial for maintaining metabolic health, and fasting, when approached sensibly, may contribute positively to this balance.

6. Reproductive Hormones: The Fertility Waltz:

- *Fasting's Influence:* Fasting can affect reproductive hormones in women. Prolonged or intense fasting may disrupt menstrual cycles, highlighting the importance of moderation and individualization.

- *Impact on Hormones:* Balancing fasting with considerations for reproductive health is essential to support hormonal equilibrium in both men and women.

7. Adiponectin and Inflammatory Modulation: The Inflammation Minuet:

- *Fasting's Influence:* Fasting may stimulate the release of adiponectin, an adipose tissue-derived hormone with anti-inflammatory properties.

- *Impact on Hormones:* Modulating inflammatory responses through fasting contributes to overall health, potentially reducing the risk of chronic inflammatory conditions.

8. Insulin-Like Growth Factor I (IGF-I): The Growth Harmony:

- *Fasting's Influence:* Fasting, exceptionally prolonged fasting, may reduce levels of IGF-I, a hormone associated with growth and cellular proliferation.

- *Impact on Hormones:* Modulating IGF-I levels is linked to potential benefits in cancer prevention and overall longevity.

Tips for Fasting and Hormonal Harmony:

- **Mindful Approaches:** Choose fasting methods that align with your needs, health status, and lifestyle.

- **Balance and Moderation:** Avoid prolonged or extreme fasting without supervision. Balance is critical to reaping benefits without negatively impacting hormonal equilibrium.

- **Nutrient-Dense Meals:** Breakfasts with nutrient-dense, balanced meals to support hormonal health and provide essential nutrients.

- **Individualization:** Recognize that individual responses to fasting may vary. Pay attention to your body's signals and adjust your approach accordingly.

- **Professional Guidance:** If you have pre-existing health conditions or concerns, consult with healthcare professionals or registered dietitians before adopting fasting practices.

Hormonal Responses to Fasting

Fasting sets the stage for a complex hormonal ballet within the body, orchestrating intricate responses that adapt to the rhythm of nutrient availability. As you delve into the world of fasting, let's unravel the hormonal symphony that unfolds during periods of reduced or absent food intake:

1. **Insulin and Glucagon Dance: Balancing Blood Sugar:**

- *Fasting's Influence:* As you enter a fasting state, insulin levels decrease, allowing the body to tap into stored glucose for energy. Conversely, glucagon levels rise, promoting the release of glucose from the liver.

- *Impact on Hormones:* This delicate dance between insulin and glucagon maintains blood sugar levels within a narrow range, ensuring a steady energy supply to cells.

2. **Growth Hormone Elevation: Cellular Repair Conductor:**

- *Fasting's Influence:* Short-term fasting, especially at night, triggers a surge in growth hormone production. Growth hormone is vital in cellular repair, metabolism, and preserving lean muscle mass.

- *Impact on Hormones:* Elevated growth hormone levels during fasting contribute to fat utilization, cellular rejuvenation, and overall metabolic balance.

3. **Cortisol Fluctuations: The Stress Response Pas de Deux:**

- *Fasting's Influence:* During the initial stages of fasting, cortisol levels may increase. This is a natural response to the stress of reduced food intake, contributing to the mobilization of energy stores.

- *Impact on Hormones:* While moderate cortisol elevation is part of the body's adaptive response, prolonged or intense fasting may lead to sustained high cortisol levels, potentially impacting stress response and hormonal equilibrium.

4. Leptin and Ghrelin Dialogue: The Appetite Ballet:

- *Fasting's Influence:* Fasting patterns balance leptin (satiety hormone) and ghrelin (hunger hormone). Leptin levels decrease, signaling to the brain that energy stores are being utilized, while ghrelin levels increase, promoting hunger.

- *Impact on Hormones:* This intricate dialogue between leptin and ghrelin regulates appetite, promoting a sense of fullness during eating and readiness for nourishment.

5. Thyroid Hormones Dance: Metabolic Symphony:

- *Fasting's Influence:* Short-term intermittent fasting has been studied for its potential impact on thyroid hormones. While thyroid hormone levels may decrease during fasting, it's often a transient and adaptive response.

- *Impact on Hormones:* Balancing the thyroid hormones is crucial for maintaining metabolic health, and fasting, when approached sensibly, may contribute positively to this balance.

6. Adiponectin Elevation: The Anti-Inflammatory Ballet:

- *Fasting's Influence:* Fasting may stimulate the release of adiponectin, an adipose tissue-derived hormone with anti-inflammatory properties.

- *Impact on Hormones:* Elevated adiponectin levels reduce systemic inflammation, potentially lowering the risk of chronic inflammatory conditions.

7. Insulin-Like Growth Factor I (IGF-I) Regulation: The Growth Harmony:

- *Fasting's Influence:* Prolonged fasting or reduced protein intake may decrease IGF-I levels, a hormone associated with growth and cellular proliferation.

- *Impact on Hormones:* Modulating IGF-I levels is linked to potential benefits in cancer prevention and overall longevity.

8. Sex Hormone Fluctuations: The Reproductive Waltz:

- *Fasting's Influence:* Fasting can affect reproductive hormones in both men and women. Prolonged or intense fasting may lead to disruptions in menstrual cycles in women.

- *Impact on Hormones:* Balancing fasting with considerations for reproductive health is essential to support hormonal equilibrium.

CHAPTER 5

Tailoring Fasting to the Female Body

Fasting, a transformative practice for many, requires a nuanced approach when tailored to the intricate rhythms of the female body. The female endocrine system is a delicate symphony of hormones, orchestrating a dance that fluctuates through various life stages. Here's a thoughtful exploration of how fasting can be harmonized with the unique needs of the female body:

1. Menstrual Cycle Awareness: The Monthly Choreography:

- *Understand the Phases:* The menstrual cycle unfolds in distinct phases, each accompanied by hormonal shifts. Consider tailoring fasting windows based on menstrual cycle phases adjusting intensity during menstruation and ovulation.

- *Gentle Adaptation:* Recognize that some women may find fasting challenging during menstruation. Listening to the body's cues and opting for more peaceful fasting approaches or modifying meal timings can provide a supportive rhythm.

2. Balancing Hormones: The Pinnacle of Well-Being:

- *Moderate Approach:* Prolonged or intense fasting may impact reproductive hormones. Opting for reasonable fasting windows and avoiding extremes can contribute to hormonal balance without disrupting the delicate dance of estrogen and progesterone.

- *Consider Individual Variability:* Each woman's hormonal landscape is unique. Pay attention to individual responses, and be open to adjusting fasting patterns based on personal experiences.

3. Nourishment during Fasting: The Essential Nutrient Waltz:

- *Prioritize Nutrient-Dense Meals:* Fasting periods should be followed by meals rich in essential nutrients. Nourishing the body with balanced and nutrient-dense foods supports overall well-being and mitigates the risk of nutrient deficiencies.

- *Emphasize Micro and Macro Nutrients:* Ensure that fasting does not compromise the intake of essential micronutrients and macronutrients crucial for hormonal health, bone density, and overall vitality.

4. Individualization and Personalization: The Key to Empowerment:

- *Unique Responses:* Women exhibit diverse responses to fasting. Embrace a personalized approach, considering age, reproductive status, and health goals.

- *Adapt as Needed:* Just as a dancer adjusts her steps to the music, adapt fasting practices based on life circumstances, stress levels, and evolving health considerations.

5. Mindful Stress Management: The Calming Ballet:

- *Cortisol Considerations:* Intermittent fasting can influence cortisol levels. Mindful stress management practices, such as meditation and gentle exercise, can complement fasting and promote a balanced stress response.

- *Prioritize Relaxation:* Recognize the importance of rest, especially during fasting. Adequate sleep and stress reduction contribute to hormonal equilibrium.

6. Consultation and Support: The Guiding Ensemble:

- *Professional Guidance:* Seeking advice from healthcare professionals or registered dietitians is invaluable. Their expertise can help tailor fasting practices to individual health profiles and address specific concerns.

- *Community Connection:* Joining a supportive community of women practicing fasting can provide shared insights, experiences, and encouragement. Collective wisdom fosters empowerment.

As women navigate the terrain of fasting, it's crucial to approach the practice with respect for the intricacies of the female body. By weaving together the threads of menstrual cycle awareness, hormonal balance, nutrient-rich nourishment, individualization, stress management, and professional guidance, fasting becomes a tailored and empowering journey for women. May it be a dance of harmony, fostering well-being, and celebrating the unique strength of the female body.

Hormonal Considerations for Fasting

Hormones, the messengers of physiological harmony, play a central role in how the body responds to periods of nutrient scarcity. Here's a thoughtful exploration of the hormonal considerations for fasting:

I. Insulin and Glucagon Duet: Blood Sugar Choreography:

- *Fasting's Influence:* During fasting, insulin levels decrease, prompting the body to utilize stored glucose for energy. Simultaneously, glucagon rises, releasing glucose from the liver into the bloodstream.

- *Impact on Hormones:* This delicate interplay ensures a steady supply of glucose, maintaining blood sugar levels within a narrow range.

2. Growth Hormone Elevation: The Cellular Repair Sonata:

- *Fasting's Influence:* Short-term fasting stimulates a surge in growth hormone production. Growth hormone is instrumental in cellular repair, muscle preservation, and metabolic balance.

- *Impact on Hormones:* Elevated growth hormone levels during fasting contribute to using stored fat for energy, supporting fat loss and overall metabolic health.

3. Cortisol Fluctuations: The Stress Response Pas de Deux:

- *Fasting's Influence:* The initial stages of fasting may lead to a temporary increase in cortisol levels. This is a natural response to the stress of reduced food intake, mobilizing energy stores.

- *Impact on Hormones:* While moderate cortisol elevation is part of the body's adaptive response, prolonged or intense fasting may lead to sustained high cortisol levels, potentially impacting stress response and hormonal equilibrium.

4. Leptin and Ghrelin Dialogue: The Appetite Ballet:

- *Fasting's Influence:* Fasting patterns balance leptin (satiety hormone) and ghrelin (hunger hormone). Leptin levels decrease, signaling to the brain that energy stores are being utilized, while ghrelin levels increase, promoting hunger.

- *Impact on Hormones:* This intricate dialogue between leptin and ghrelin regulates appetite, promoting a sense of fullness during eating and readiness for nourishment.

5. Thyroid Hormones Dance: Metabolic Symphony:

- *Fasting's Influence:* Short-term intermittent fasting has been studied for its potential impact on thyroid hormones.

While thyroid hormone levels may decrease during fasting, it's often a transient and adaptive response.

- *Impact on Hormones:* Balancing the thyroid hormones is crucial for maintaining metabolic health, and fasting, when approached sensibly, may contribute positively to this balance.

6. Adiponectin Elevation: The Anti-Inflammatory Ballet:

- *Fasting's Influence:* Fasting may stimulate the release of adiponectin, an adipose tissue-derived hormone with anti-inflammatory properties.

- *Impact on Hormones:* Elevated adiponectin levels reduce systemic inflammation, potentially lowering the risk of chronic inflammatory conditions.

7. Insulin-Like Growth Factor I (IGF-I) Regulation: The Growth Harmony:

- *Fasting's Influence:* Prolonged fasting or reduced protein intake may decrease IGF-I levels, a hormone associated with growth and cellular proliferation.

- *Impact on Hormones:* Modulating IGF-I levels is linked to potential benefits in cancer prevention and overall longevity.

8. Sex Hormone Fluctuations: The Reproductive Waltz:

- *Fasting's Influence:* Fasting can affect reproductive hormones in both men and women. Prolonged or intense fasting may lead to disruptions in menstrual cycles in women.

- *Impact on Hormones:* Balancing fasting with considerations for reproductive health is essential to support hormonal equilibrium.

Menstrual Cycle and Fasting

The menstrual cycle is a rhythmic dance of hormonal fluctuations that requires a delicate and mindful approach when considering fasting practices. Tailoring fasting to the menstrual cycle phases can support women in fostering overall well-being. Let's explore the nuanced interplay between menstrual cycles and fasting:

1. Menstrual Phase: Embracing Gentle Nourishment:

- *Understanding the Phase:* The menstrual phase is marked by the shedding of the uterine lining. During this time, women may experience fatigue and lower energy levels.

- *Fasting Considerations:* Opting for gentler fasting methods or extending the eating window can provide the body with essential nutrients and energy, supporting a more nurturing approach during menstruation.

2. Follicular Phase: Energizing Renewal:

- *Understanding the Phase:* The follicular phase follows menstruation and is characterized by a rise in estrogen levels. Energy levels typically increase during this phase.

- *Fasting Considerations:* Women may find this phase conducive to more extended fasting periods, as increased energy levels align with the body's natural rhythms.

3. Ovulatory Phase: Fertility and Vitality:

- *Understanding the Phase:* Ovulation, marked by the release of an egg, occurs in the middle of the menstrual cycle. Hormones like estrogen peak during this phase.

- *Fasting Considerations:* This phase may suit balanced fasting practices, aligning with the body's vitality and metabolic peaks.

4. Luteal Phase: Hormonal Ebb and Flow:

- *Understanding the Phase:* The luteal phase follows ovulation and precedes menstruation. Progesterone levels rise, and some women may experience mood changes or cravings.

- *Fasting Considerations:* Adopting a mindful approach to fasting, potentially with shorter or less intense fasting periods, can support hormonal balance during this phase.

Practical Insights for Fasting and Menstrual Harmony:

- **Cycle Tracking:** Awareness of menstrual cycle phases can guide fasting practices. Many apps are available to help track menstrual cycles and identify different stages.

- **Individual Variability:** Women's experiences with fasting during the menstrual cycle vary. Pay attention to your body's signals and adjust fasting approaches based on individual responses.

- **Hydration and Nutrition:** Prioritize hydration and nourishing, nutrient-dense foods throughout the menstrual cycle. Proper hydration and balanced nutrition are foundational for well-being.

- **Adaptation over Rigidity:** Consider a flexible approach to fasting, adapting your practices based on how you feel during different phases of the menstrual cycle.

- **Professional Guidance:** Consult with healthcare professionals or registered dietitians, especially if you have specific health concerns or if fasting practices impact your menstrual cycle adversely.

Fasting during Pregnancy and Lactation

Pregnancy and lactation are profound life stages that demand careful consideration of nutritional needs and overall well-being. While fasting practices can offer benefits, they also pose potential risks during these critical periods. Let's explore the nuanced considerations surrounding fasting during pregnancy and lactation:

Fasting During Pregnancy: A Gentle Approach:

1. **Nourishing the Growing Life:**

   - *Critical Nutrient Demands:* Pregnancy demands increased nutrient intake for the developing fetus. Fasting, exceedingly prolonged or intense fasting, may compromise the essential nutrients required for fetal growth and development.

   - *Potential Risks:* Fasting during pregnancy carries the risk of inadequate calorie and nutrient intake, which can impact the health of both the mother and the developing baby.

2. **Hormonal Stability and Growth:**

   - *Hormonal Considerations:* Pregnancy hormones play a crucial role in maintaining a stable environment for fetal development. Sudden changes in nutrient availability, such as those induced by fasting, can disrupt this delicate hormonal balance.

- *Cautionary Note:* Fasting practices that might induce stress on the body should be cautiously approached during pregnancy to avoid potential complications.

3. **Professional Guidance:**

- *Consultation is Crucial:* Pregnant individuals should consult with healthcare providers, including obstetricians and dietitians, before considering fasting practices. Individual health status and pregnancy-specific factors should guide decisions.

Fasting During Lactation: Balancing Nutrition for Both:

1. **Nutrient Demands for Breastfeeding:**

- *Increased Caloric Needs:* Lactation demands additional energy and nutrients to support milk production. Fasting practices that compromise calorie and nutrient intake can impact the quality and quantity of breast milk.

- *Potential Dehydration:* Extended fasting without proper hydration may lead to dehydration, affecting milk supply.

2. **Hormonal Stability for Milk Production:**

- *Hormonal Influences:* Hormones like prolactin play a central role in milk production. Fasting-induced stress may interfere with the hormonal balance needed for optimal lactation.

- *Maintaining a Stable Routine:* Stable and consistent nutritional intake supports hormonal equilibrium for sustained milk production.

3. **Professional Guidance:**

   - *Consult with Experts:* Lactating individuals should seek guidance from healthcare professionals, including lactation consultants and dietitians. Individualized advice can ensure that fasting practices do not compromise maternal and infant well-being.

Practical Insights and Caution:

1. **Hydration and Balanced Nutrition:**

   - *Foundational Principles:* Adequate hydration and balanced nutrition are foundational during pregnancy and lactation. Fasting practices should prioritize meeting these essential needs.

2. **Mindful Approaches:**

   - *Flexibility and Adaptation:* If considering fasting during these periods, adopt a flexible and adaptive approach. The mother and child's well-being should take precedence over fasting goals.

3. **Listening to the Body:**

   - *Individual Responses:* Pay close attention to individual responses. If fasting induces fatigue, dizziness, or any adverse effects, it's crucial to reconsider the approach.

4. **Cultural and Religious Considerations:**

- *Respect Individual Beliefs:* Some cultures or religions may have fasting practices embedded in traditions. In such cases, it's essential to integrate these practices with careful attention to nutritional needs and consult with healthcare providers.

Fasting during pregnancy and lactation necessitates a cautious and informed approach. The primary focus should be on nourishing the mother and the developing child. Consultation with healthcare professionals is paramount, ensuring that any fasting practices align with the unique needs of these transformative life stages. May this journey be one of balance, nourishment, and maternal well-being.

Creating a Personalized Fasting Plan

Creating a personalized fasting plan involves self-discovery, mindful choices, and a commitment to overall well-being. Here's a guide to help you craft a fasting plan tailored to your unique needs, goals, and lifestyle:

I. Understanding Your Goals:

- *Clarify Intentions:* Define the purpose of your fasting journey. Understanding your goals will shape your approach, whether it's for weight management, metabolic health, or spiritual reasons.

- *Long-Term Vision:* Consider your long-term vision for well-being. A sustainable fasting plan aligns with your broader health goals.

2. Assessing Your Health Status:

- *Consultation with Professionals:* Before starting any fasting plan, consult healthcare professionals. This is especially crucial if you have pre-existing health conditions or are taking medications.

- *Nutritional Assessment:* Evaluate your current nutritional status. Understanding your baseline helps tailor a fasting plan that meets your nutrient needs.

3. Identifying Your Fasting Window:

- *Daily or Intermittent Fasting:* Decide on the duration of your fasting window. Options include daily fasting (e.g., 16/8 method) or intermittent fasting (e.g., 5:2 form).

- *Consider Lifestyle:* Align your fasting window with your daily routine and preferences. Choose a pattern that seamlessly integrates with your lifestyle.

4. Choosing Fasting Methods:

- *Explore Variations:* There are various fasting methods, such as water fasting, juice fasting, or time-restricted eating. Choose a way that resonates with you and suits your health goals.

- *Experimentation:* Be open to experimenting with different methods. Your body's response may vary; finding what works best for you may involve trial and error.

5. Listening to Your Body:

- *Body Signals:* Pay attention to your body's signals during fasting. If you feel tired, dizzy, or experience other adverse effects, it might be an indicator to adjust your fasting approach.

- *Adaptability:* Your body's needs may change over time. Be adaptable and willing to modify your fasting plan based on evolving circumstances.

6. Incorporating Nutrient-Rich Meals:

- *Balanced Nutrition:* Break your fasts with nutrient-dense, balanced meals. Prioritize a variety of whole foods to ensure you meet your nutritional requirements.

- *Hydration:* Stay well-hydrated during fasting periods. Water, herbal teas, and other non-caloric beverages contribute to overall hydration.

7. Mindful Eating Practices:

- *Conscious Choices:* When you eat, practice mindfulness. Be present during meals, savoring each bite. This promotes a healthy relationship with food.

- *Avoiding Bingeing:* Be cautious of overeating when breaking your fast. Gradually reintroduce food to prevent digestive discomfort.

8. Monitoring Progress and Adjusting:

- *Regular Check-Ins:* Periodically assess your progress. Monitor how your body responds to fasting and make adjustments as needed.

- *Celebrate Milestones:* Acknowledge and celebrate achievements, whether they relate to your health goals, improved energy levels, or other positive outcomes.

9. Incorporating Holistic Wellness Practices:

- *Complementary Practices:* Integrate holistic wellness practices into your routine, such as regular exercise, stress management, and sufficient sleep.

- *Holistic Approach:* Fasting is just one component of overall well-being. A holistic approach that considers physical, mental, and emotional aspects enhances the effectiveness of your plan.

10. Seeking Support and Community:

- *Community Engagement:* Joining a community of individuals with similar fasting goals can provide support, insights, and motivation.

- *Professional Guidance:* Consider working with a registered dietitian or healthcare provider for personalized advice and support.

Self-Help Questions

1. **Clarifying Intentions:**

   - What is my primary goal in exploring fasting?

   - How do I envision fasting contributing to my overall well-being?

2. **Reflecting on Readiness:**

   - Am I mentally and emotionally prepared to embark on a fasting journey?

   - What aspects of my life support or challenge my readiness for this exploration?

3. **Understanding Personal Health:**

   - Have I consulted with healthcare professionals to assess my health status?

   - What are my specific health goals, and how might fasting align with them?

4. **Exploring Motivations:**

   - What motivates me to incorporate fasting into my life?

   - How do I envision my life changing or improving through this practice?

5. **Setting Realistic Expectations:**

   - What are my expectations for the outcomes of fasting?

- Have I considered both short-term and long-term expectations realistically?

6. **Assessing Lifestyle Compatibility:**

   - How can I integrate fasting into my daily or weekly routine?

   - What potential challenges might arise, and how can I navigate them?

7. **Acknowledging Individuality:**

   - What unique aspects of my lifestyle, preferences, or health history should influence my fasting approach?

   - How can I tailor my fasting plan to align with my needs?

8. **Checking Mindful Engagement:**

   - How mindful am I about my relationship with food?

   - Can I practice mindfulness during meals, especially when fast-breaking?

9. **Monitoring Progress:**

   - What benchmarks can I set to measure the success of my fasting journey?

   - How frequently will I check in with myself to assess progress and make adjustments?

10. **Cultivating Holistic Wellness:**

   - In addition to fasting, what other holistic practices can complement my well-being?

- How can I create a balanced lifestyle beyond fasting to support my physical, mental, and emotional health?

11. **Building a Support System:**

    - Do I have a support system or community to share my journey with?

    - How can I seek professional guidance or engage with others with similar goals?

12. **Understanding Hormonal Health:**

    - What is my current understanding of hormonal health, and how do hormones affect my well-being?

    - What aspects of hormonal balance do I hope to learn more about in this chapter?

13. **Awareness of Hormonal Impact:**

    - How conscious am I of the potential impact of hormonal balance on my physical and mental health?

    - In what ways do I currently observe or experience the effects of hormonal fluctuations in my life?

14. **Personalizing Hormonal Wellness:**

    - To what extent do I believe that hormonal wellness is a personalized journey?

    - How open am I to tailoring practices to support my unique hormonal needs?

15. **Exploring Historical Perspectives:**

- What historical perspectives or cultural influences have shaped my understanding of feminine wellness and hormonal balance?

- How might historical views impact my current approach to health and wellness?

16. **Modern Insights and Knowledge:**

- How updated is my knowledge about modern perspectives on feminine wellness and hormonal health?

- What new insights or information am I hoping to gain from this chapter?

17. **Valuing Hormonal Balance:**

- On a scale from 1 to 10, how much importance do I currently place on maintaining hormonal balance?

- What factors influence the value I attribute to hormonal well-being?

18. **Connecting Physical and Mental Health:**

- Am I aware of the interconnectedness between hormonal balance, physical health, and mental well-being?

- In what ways do I see the link between hormonal health and my overall vitality?

19. **Identifying Hormonal Challenges:**

- Have I identified specific hormonal challenges or concerns in my life?

- How do these challenges manifest, and how do they impact my daily life?

20. Setting Hormonal Wellness Goals:

- What goals do I hope to achieve by focusing on hormonal wellness?

- How will achieving these goals positively influence different aspects of my life?

21. Evaluating Lifestyle Choices:

- To what extent do my current lifestyle choices align with hormonal health?

- What adjustments, if any, am I willing to make to support hormonal balance?

22. Curiosity and Learning:

- How curious am I about the intricate details of the endocrine system and hormone function?

- What specific aspects of hormonal science am I excited to learn more about?

23. Hormone Production and Release:

- What role does hormone production and release play in maintaining homeostasis within the body?

- How does the timing and quantity of hormone release contribute to overall health?

24. Hormones and Their Functions:

- Can I identify some essential hormones and their functions in the body?

- In what ways do these hormones impact various physiological processes?

25. Essential Hormones in Women:

- Do I understand the hormones that are particularly relevant to women's health?

- How do these hormones influence different stages of a woman's life?

26. Interactions and Feedback Mechanisms:

- Am I aware of the intricate feedback mechanisms that regulate hormonal balance?

- How do these feedback loops contribute to the body's ability to maintain equilibrium?

27. Connecting Hormones to Health:

- In what ways do hormonal imbalances manifest in physical and mental health symptoms?

- How might understanding these connections empower me to make informed health choices?

Get a sheet of paper and answer these questions on your day-to-day activities.